DAVE DOWLING

MOB 07770532337

ASSESSING COMMAND AND CONTROL EFFECTIVENESS

Human Factors in Defence

Series Editors:
Dr Don Harris, Managing Director of HFI Solutions Ltd, UK
Professor Neville Stanton, Chair in Human Factors at the
University of Southampton, UK
Dr Eduardo Salas, University of Central Florida, USA

Human factors is key to enabling today's armed forces to implement their vision to "produce battle-winning people and equipment that are fit for the challenge of today, ready for the tasks of tomorrow and capable of building for the future" (source: UK MoD). Modern armed forces fulfil a wider variety of roles thanever before. In addition to defending sovereign territory and prosecuting armed conflicts, military personnel are engaged in homeland defence and in undertaking peacekeeping operations and delivering humanitarian aid right across the world.

This requires top class personnel, trained to the highest standards in the use offirst class equipment. The military has long recognised that good human factors is essential if these aims are to be achieved.

The defence sector is far and away the largest employer of human factors personnel across the globe and is the largest funder of basic and applied research. Much of this research is applicable to a wide audience, not just the military; this series aims to give readers access to some of this high quality work.

Ashgate's *Human Factors in Defence* series comprises of specially commissioned books from internationally recognised experts in the field. They provide in-depth, authoritative accounts of key human factors issues being addressed by the defence industry across the world.

Assessing Command and Control Effectiveness
Dealing with a Changing World

Edited by

PETER BERGGREN
FOI, Swedish Defence Research Agency, Sweden

STAFFAN NÄHLINDER
FOI, Swedish Defence Research Agency, Sweden

ERLAND SVENSSON
Formerly FOI, Swedish Defence Research Agency, Sweden

ASHGATE

Published by
Ashgate Publishing Limited
Wey Court East
Union Road
Farnham
Surrey, GU9 7PT
England

Ashgate Publishing Company
110 Cherry Street
Suite 3-1
Burlington, VT 05401-3818
USA

www.ashgate.com

British Library Cataloguing in Publication Data
A catalogue record for this book is available from the British Library

The Library of Congress has cataloged the printed edition as follows:
Assessing command and control effectiveness : dealing with a changing world / [edited] by Peter Berggren, Staffan Ndhlinder and Erland Svensson.
    pages cm -- (Human factors in defence) Includes bibliographical references and index.
  ISBN 978-1-4724-3694-8 (hardback) -- ISBN 978-1-4724-3695-5 (ebook) -- ISBN 978-1-4724-3696-2 (epub) 1. Command and control systems--Evaluation. 2. Command and control systems--Research--Methodology. I. Berggren, Peter, 1971- editor of compilation. II. Ndhlinder, Staffan, 1971- editor of compilation. III. Svensson, Erland, 1945- editor of compilation. IV. Series: Human factors in defence.
  UB212.A88 2014
  355.3'3041--dc23

2014003386

ISBN 9781472436948 (hbk)
ISBN 9781472436955 (ebk – PDF)
ISBN 9781472436962 (ebk – ePUB)

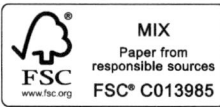

Printed in the United Kingdom by Henry Ling Limited, at the Dorset Press, Dorchester, DT1 1HD

Contents

List of Figures

List of Tables

List of Contributors

Editors

Peter Berggren is a senior scientist at FOI, the Swedish Defence Research Agency. He holds an MSc in cognitive science from the University of Linköping. His principal research interests lie in measures and analysis of teamwork effectiveness, decision-making and command and control performance assessments. Peter has worked with human factors research since 1998. He has studied fighter pilots, individual soldiers, tank commanders, brigade staffs, as well as civil crisis management and emergency response. By participating in military exercises as a scientist, Peter has a long experience of working closely with the military in field-experimentation-like situations. Peter is a project manager for an Armed Forces project on assessing command and control effectiveness.

Staffan Nählinder is a senior scientist at FOI, the Swedish Defence Research Agency. He holds an MSc in psychology and statistics from the University of Uppsala and a PhD in human–machine interaction from the University of Linköping. His principal research interests concern training, decision-making, performance assessment, mental workload and situation awareness. He has worked with human factors research since 1998. Among other things he has worked with various psychophysiological measures to assess mental workload in both military and civil pilots in both simulated and real flight. Staffan has also worked with transfer of training questions in military training facilities.

Erland Svensson, PhD, is retired director of research at the Swedish Defence Research Agency (FOI) and professor emeritus at the University of Linköping. He is former director of the Department of Man–System Interaction (FOI-MSI) and of the Institute of Aviation Medicine, Linköping. His research includes measurements of mental workload, situational awareness, operative performance, modelling and simulation. Erland has been the Swedish Partnership for Peace representative for the NATO Research and Technology Organisation (RTO) Human Factors and Medicine Panel. He has been national point of contact for cooperative activities between the US Air Force Research Laboratory, the Netherlands Organization for Applied Scientific Research (TNO), the UK Defence Science and Technology Laboratory and Defence Research and Development Canada, and governmental expert in the European Defence Agency (EDA). Erland has been a member of the Royal Aeronautical Society, London, of the board of the Swedish Society for Human Factors, and he is a member of the Swedish Society for MPs and

Scientists (RIFO). He has been secretary of the board of the Swedish Aeronautical and Naval Medical Association. In his retired position, Erland is developing techniques for the measurement of dynamic processes at FOI and he is associated with the Department of Cardiology, University of Linköping, in research on psychophysiological modelling.

Contributors

Magdalena Granåsen works as a scientist at the Swedish Defence Research Agency. She has a Masters in cognitive science at Linköping University, Sweden. She is a PhD student in informatics. Her research is mainly focused on aspects of team information sharing. She has lately studied communication through social media during crisis response, sharing of information between civilian and military actors in international peace operations and communication between military actors during combat. Furthermore, she has conducted research concerning military command and control systems and methodology. As a reserve officer in the Swedish Army, she is familiar with military procedures and participates regularly in military training and exercises.

Björn Johansson (associate professor, PhD in cognitive systems) is a deputy research director at the Swedish Defence Research Agency as well as an assistant professor at Linköping University. Björn's research focus is cognitive systems, resilience engineering, command and control, the temporal characteristics of control tasks and communication. He has worked in several different projects concerned with crisis management and information technology, traffic and air traffic management, as well as command and control systems. Björn's work at Linköping University involves teaching and supervision in the cognitive science programme. He has also been employed at Combitech AB and Saab Security, performing various conceptual work concerning crisis management systems.

Jenny Marklund has a Bachelor of Arts degree in cognitive science from Skövde University, Sweden. During her 11 years at FOI she has mainly conducted research in military command and control settings studying different human factors issues. Recently, her work has focused on developing methods for improving the military lessons-learned process from international operations. She is the author and co-author of many international peer-reviewed publications.

Dr Arne Norlander is Research and Development Director at the Swedish Armed Forces Defence Staff. He directs research in modelling, simulation and aerospace technologies, and leads international research cooperation between the Armed Forces and academic institutions. Arne also oversees the Swedish military postgraduate education programme. Arne holds Masters, Licentiate and Doctoral degrees from Linköping University and the Stockholm Royal Institute of Technology, and he is a graduate of the Swedish National Defence College. Arne's research focus is in computerized automation, human–machine interaction, control theory, mathematical modelling, cybernetics, cognitive systems engineering, innovation management, team decision-making and team training.

Paul V. Pearce is a principal analyst within the Defence Science and Technology Laboratory of the United Kingdom. His research focus is on command and control, specifically on the modelling and simulation of command and control within the land environment to support force development and procurement decision-making within the UK MoD. More recently, he has been the UK lead on the NATO SAS-085 research task group looking at command and control agility. He is a Fellow of the Operational Research Society, a chartered engineer within the British Computer Society and has recently gained a Diploma in Psychology from the Open University. He is the author and co-author of a number of publications within the command and control area.

Carin Rencrantz is project manager and analyst at the Swedish Civil Contingencies Agency (MSB). Her work focuses on developing, implementing and evaluating methods to conduct cross-sector exercises. The overall aim of the work is to improve the ability of individual organizations and society to handle emergencies.

Peter Thunholm has a PhD in cognitive psychology and is Professor of War Studies, especially operational art and tactics, at the Swedish National Defence College in Stockholm. He is also an associate professor of psychology at Stockholm University and a lieutenant colonel in the Swedish Armed Forces. Peter's primary research focused on military planning and decision-making and he developed a model of military tactical planning that is now doctrine in the Swedish Armed Forces. More recently, his research focused on command and control of military operations. He is the author and co-author of several international peer-reviewed publications.

Jiri Trnka is a scientist at the Swedish Defence Research Agency. He has a PhD in informatics (2009). His research focuses on information support for collaborative command and control in emergency and crisis response operations. He has participated in a number of projects concerned with command and control, decision support systems, simulation and training. Besides research he has expertise in the areas of planning, execution and evaluation of major crisis and emergency management exercises.

Per Wikberg has a PhD in cognitive systems and works as a senior scientist at the Swedish Defence Research Agency. The scope of his research has been on research methodology in practical settings. His research has been undertaken in a large variety of organizations in the context of studies focusing on a wide variety of issues such as decision-making, situation awareness, access to real-time information, automated sensor information processing, delegation of command and control responsibility and comparison of different ways to present a situational picture.

Rogier Woltjer is a senior scientist at the Swedish Defence Research Agency (FOI). He obtained a PhD in cognitive systems (2009) from Linköping University, Sweden. His research focuses on the development of new concepts and methods in safety, security, human factors and resilience, in complex socio-technical work systems such as emergency and crisis response and air traffic management. His research and work in industry has addressed training, decision support, command and control, risk analysis, incident investigation and safety management.

Forewords

The authors have provided a significant contribution to what the greater human factors community calls 'human systems technologies'. It has been well over a decade since the first meaningful papers and discussions on how the human functions in our new, complex world of multiple, unexpected cognitive stimuli. The areas of human systems technologies have, over the years, had a variety of specialties on which they focused. From Paul Fitts and human engineering (HE) or ergonomics, to human factors engineering (HFE) and human systems integration (HSI), and now we are experiencing a more inclusive human systems (HS) technology. Throughout this sequence we see the growth and maturation of our knowledge and the focus of new application opportunities. Thus we seem to have gone from (human) engineering design to (human) systems integration and most recently it seems that the inclusion of cognitive systems is a foundation of our future for the integration of humans and systems.

This book provides a significant review of where our science and technology innovations are leading us. The neural science backbone succinctly explains the foundational knowledge base of how our neural–cognitive system can deal with the emergence and understanding of innovation. I applaud the editors and authors of this book for recognizing that the use of cognitive and decision science's breakthroughs is indeed how to leverage the innovations provided by today's and most certainly tomorrow's emerging computer-based human interface technologies. The uses of modelling and simulation capabilities to explore the complex and often underappreciated process of complex decision-making are well expressed in these chapters. This book clearly discusses cognitive processes in terms of tactical decision-making. However, it is only a small step towards more strategic and multifaceted applications. All through this book one finds significant data and references to support new and expanded opportunities for the operation and maintenance (sustained expertise) related to education and training. While the examples are based on tactical systems with mission outcomes, the potential vulnerability of not following the input and resultant outcomes can have devastating results to mission effectiveness. This book and many of its references should be used to mentor those new to, or currently active in, the design of complex and successful decision-making systems. This is a well-structured discussion of the history and future for where and how neural–cognitive science and theory will be able to impact our future design of manned and autonomous systems. Having been a USA delegate to NATO's Research and Technology Organization, and currently being a delegate to the Science and Technology Organization's Human Factors and Medical Panel, I continue to be impressed with Sweden's technology contributions to our global knowledge base. As I read these chapters, it was easy to envision how using these findings can significantly impact the success of our alliance's government organizations. The NATO Human Factors and Medical Panel, to which I devote a lot of attention, is constantly striving to embrace those human systems technologies which will have a significant impact on training and human effectiveness in the decades to come. It is within our alliances that we have to constantly and quickly deal with increasingly complex multicultural environments that include new processes, all with the goal of improving the overall effectiveness of the synergy of people and systems. However, we know that as the complexity of our human–systems environment increases we need the agility to explore more alternatives that often require non-linear innovation. This capability can now be explored earlier in the design phases, before a real tactical command and control system is built, using validated synthetic environments.

The challenge to the readers and believers in the future of applying the findings of these papers, therefore, is to try one's design philosophy out first in a synthetic environment designed to allow meaningful assessment of human–system performance and to investigate how performance varies as environmental constraints *and* mission goals change. Armed with these data, one can see a new decade where cognitive systems knowledge and technologies will spawn yet unknown opportunities for future decision-making technologies and systems.

In summary, the following chapters will significantly help one understand how the use of modelling and simulations in the human systems context can help design more complex decision-making interfaces at equal or reduced cost with equal or better operational effectiveness.

Paul Chatelier

———

Command and control has changed considerably since 1990. Think of network technology allowing information to be shared faster, over larger areas, and independent of hierarchical lines. Think of the change from the large, organic unit operations to small-unit operations composed of coalition military, taking cooperation to an unprecedented level of integration. Think of the change from military–military confrontations to 'war amongst the people … with civilians around, against civilians, in defence of civilians' (General Sir Rupert Smith). Think of the growing coordinated interaction and cooperation with governmental and non-governmental agencies using comprehensive instruments to improve security and safety conditions for the people.

For me, it took several years before I began to realize the impact of changing world on command and control beyond just being better networked. The profound events of 1994 (Rwanda) and 1995 (Srebrenica) marked the ambivalent position of military operations in uncertain and fuzzy political conditions. The 'Human in Command' conferences (in 1998: 'Exploring the Modern Military Experience'; and 2000: 'Peace Support Operations') were the first to focus on the human dimensions of command and control. This was initially from the perspective of the military entity, but recently the scope broadened to the ecosystem of multiple actors, including the military, in the operation area. With several international partners we started to study 'command team effectiveness'. We saw the team, networked with other teams, as the essential unit of command and control. This work was done in the context of trilateral cooperation between Sweden, the Netherlands and Canada ('Command in NEC'), and in task groups of the NATO Science and Technology Human Factors and Medicine Panel ('Command Team Effectiveness – CTEF').

Two of the editors of this book, Erland Svensson and Peter Berggren, were among the partners digging deeper in the new realities of command and control. We learned that operational practice developed faster than conceptual or laboratory studies could deliver their results. We learned also that it takes substantial effort to set up a sufficiently sound assessment of the impact of teamwork, new structures and new technologies. Research 'in the wild' is needed to further our knowledge and to provide scientific guidance to operational practitioners. The challenge is how to do that research, given the limitations of operational practice: too much rigour is not practical, but too little rigour brings little value to the operator. This should be understood and appreciated by researchers and operators.

Berggren, Nählinder and Svensson took up the challenge, and, together with researchers from the Swedish Defence Research Agency and the Swedish Defence College, continued to develop and apply practical approaches to assessment. How to develop a systematic approach to operational assessment delivering accountable value is one of the challenges addressed in this book. The book brings together approaches and insights, which is of high relevance for (applied) researchers and for operational practitioners.

Peter Essens, PhD
Principal Scientist, Behavioural and Societal Sciences,
Netherlands Organization for Applied Scientific Research (TNO)
Member NATO Human Factors and Medicine Panel,
Area Leader Human Effectiveness

Preface

Command and control is increasingly important in our world, with high demands for interoperability, agility and international cooperation. However, for quite some time, methods for assessing command and control effectiveness have not kept up with the demands and requirements of a rapidly changing world.

During the last decade, worldwide interest in command and control research has increased considerably. There have been several NATO RTO groups aimed at developing command and control research and quite a few bilateral and trilateral agreements between nations working together to boost development in this area. In Sweden, the Armed Forces aimed to develop new command and control systems, and provided researchers ample opportunities for empirical studies.

This book is a summary over central parts of the Swedish command and control research – from a human factors perspective – that has been conducted over the last decade. It is a testament of the research that has been performed and what the main themes and conclusions from this important research area are. It is a look forward, towards an unknown but quite complex and dynamic future. It is a stepping stone, looking towards the future and at the challenges of dealing with a changing world.

The intended audience for this book is researchers as well as practitioners. We believe the book can be used by researchers to develop hypotheses for investigations and as inspiration for methodological discussions. It can also be used by practitioners to expand their understanding of the research process and to learn more about how command and control can be studied. Military personnel interested in developing a better understanding of the command and control research will find new perspectives and examples in this book. We believe that researchers and practitioners in other related research fields such as crisis response and management, civil command and control and persons developing decision support systems will also find this book useful.

Most of the research presented in the book has been funded by the Swedish Armed Forces' research and development programme for science and technology.

Acknowledgements

We would first like to thank FOI, the Swedish Defence Research Agency, for providing a scientific and creative research environment. We would like to thank the Swedish Armed Forces for supporting the research and providing personnel who willingly filled out questionnaires and participated in experiments and field studies.

We would like to direct a special thanks to Mr Paul R. Chatelier for introducing us to NATO RTO research activities on performance assessment in command and control, and to Dr Peter Essens who has enabled several studies and collaborations.

We also want to acknowledge Natascha Korolija who proofread most texts and gave invaluable feedback and advice to all authors. We thank Henrik Allberg who was of great help with practical issues concerning the writing of the main part of the book.

Another acknowledgement is the many inspirational and educative environments that we have all been part of, both in terms of discussions and experiences of empirical situations.

And last, but not least, thank you Karolina, Johanna and Maud.

Chapter 1

Introduction

P. Berggren, S. Nählinder and E. Svensson

Assessing Command and Control Effectiveness –
Dealing with a Changing World

There is constant development in military command and control. New systems are developed and old systems are used in new contexts. This concerns methods, work, manning and command and control technology. There is clearly a need to have a research process to support this development. The research process should assess, analyse and communicate results to the development cycle. It should be effective, meaning it should be quick and simple, cost-effective while still being able to draw valid conclusions. Further, it should be done without disturbing the ongoing command and control work.

This book offers a description of the current state of command and control research in settings where sample sizes are small, opportunities are few and resources are limited. Special attention is given to the development of command and control research methods to meet the current and coming needs.

The purpose of command and control research is to improve the command and control process and make it more effective while still saving time and money. The research methods have to be chosen carefully to be effective and simple, yet provide results of high quality. Methodological concerns are a major consideration when working under such circumstances. Further, there is often a need for a swift iterative development cycle, and thus a demand to quickly deliver results from the research process. This book explains how field research experimentation can be quick, simple and effective, even though sample sizes are small and resources are limited. In such conditions, empirical data often need to be collected using measures and procedures that are minimally intrusive.

In classical experimentation it is common to use control groups and to manipulate the conditions of interest in a controlled fashion. In the command and control setting it is difficult to design research studies using classical experimentation. The problems and situations often occur rarely, and only a few practitioners are specialized and experienced. The command and control environment is dynamic and complex and the possibilities for experimental control are few. This means that classical experimental designs are very hard to achieve, and that traditional techniques for analysis might not give a truthful or complete picture. The limits on available data require special experimental designs, procedures and statistical techniques to be applied.

This book will provide examples on how dynamic assessment can be performed, explain how dynamic situations can be assessed and analysed, explain the benefits and concerns regarding dynamic measurements and provide empirical examples and discuss differences and similarities between civil and military command and control.

The book furthers the research by showing how command and control studies can be performed in field settings characterized by dynamic and complex situations, describing how dynamic command and control situations can be assessed using dynamic methods and advanced statistical procedures, and giving examples of how the stakeholders and end users can be involved in the command and control research process and be provided with quick feedback.

Overview of the Book

After this introductory chapter, the reader will be presented with theoretical foundations for the assessment of effectiveness in the command and control domain. After that, the reader will be provided with several empirical studies of command and control effectiveness. Before the concluding chapter, a look forward is presented with ideas about agile command and control in the near future.

Analysing Tactical Cognitive Systems

Norlander describes how, in military operations and emergency management, operators and commanders must rely on distributed systems for safe and effective mission accomplishment. Tactical commanders and operators tend to encounter violent threats, and critical demands are frequently imposed on cognitive capacity and reaction time. In the future, decisions will be made in situations where operational and system characteristics are non-linear, that is, 'small' actions or decisions may have serious, even irreversible, consequences for an entire mission. Such situations, in short, possess distinct, complex and dynamic properties.

The objective of this research is to integrate relevant, effective methods and tools that improve command and control procedures, as well as the design of future command and control systems. A broad research approach is pursued and theoretical and practical perspectives combined to discover novel and effective ways to accomplish the objective. Experiences from this work make it possible to develop theories, methods and tools for modelling and analysis to prevent failures and accidents in precarious time-critical systems control in emergency response operations and military missions. Critical skills of individual operators and teams, mission resource management, decision-making and overall unit performance constitute the primary fields of study.

This chapter reports research work which develops an integrated approach to information-centred systems analysis. This approach, in turn, supports future command and control systems development, as well as future research on related topics.

Designing Case Studies Using a Systems Analysis Approach

Wikberg explains that in development projects, it might be difficult to fully apply the experimental method. Combining complex systems is not always possible in a laboratory setting and too much control means losing the dynamics of real operations. This chapter outlines an approach to designing case studies based on systems analysis. The main argument is that a systems analysis approach makes it possible to more efficiently make advances in a development process. The concepts of, and practical implications from, case studies and systems analysis are elaborated. Several issues are raised. First, the problem of defining which factors to include and how to select corresponding empirical indicators is addressed. This is suggested that this can be handled by comparing common and unique variations between information sources with a preliminary analysis of the system analysis subject. Second, it is recommended to avoid formalized procedures for the system analysis. Third, case studies do not necessarily aim at generalized knowledge valid in 'all' relevant situations. Thus, the validity of the case study should be assessed in the context of the aim of the development process. Finally, the question whether case studies qualify to be labelled 'science' is raised. The position is that each case study should be judged individually. Carefully designed studies are as important in a practical project as in science.

Dynamic Measures of Effectiveness in Command and Control

Svensson and Nählinder point out that classical experiment designs and statistical techniques are great tools in situations where there is control over the experiment conditions, and where the focus of attention is analysis of (static) differences between two or more conditions. When conducting research in a command and control setting, on the other hand, classical experimental procedures and statistical techniques must be deemed insufficient. A command and control environment is dynamic and complex, and the possibilities for experimental control are few. Here, the aim is to understand dynamic relationships between variables. Technical systems and operators (and teams of operators) interact over time to reach a shared goal. Furthermore, focused variables are usually abstract. For instance, in the development and operational evaluation of command and control systems, some important variables are mental workload (information load), situational awareness (situation assessment, understanding, attention) and aspects of individual and team performance (decision-making). Such variables all change over time as a function of both external and internal factors. Statistical measures adapted to these situations are therefore obviously needed. Dynamic processes and changes over periods of time are in focus, and dynamic measures in terms of repeated, or time series, measures are called for. Dynamic measures generate information that cannot be made available using traditional experiment designs and questionnaires. By means of time series measures, relationships between dynamic changes of variables (cross-correlations) and their ability to predict future events can be estimated.

Organizational Agility – An Overview

In this chapter Johansson and Pearce present a model of organizational agility based on a review of relevant research material. The theories and views presented in the model could be used to inform current and future research activities. The model is based on four themes. First, there is a theme of awareness or the ability to anticipate some effect on an organization: being proactive. Secondly, there is a theme of resilience and delivery of an appropriate response from a range of available response options: being reactive. Thirdly, there is a theme stressing continual organizational learning, which is also synonymous with being reflexive and adaptable. Fourthly, there is a theme concerning failure of an organization to respond effectively and thereby being able to absorb shock from an unexpected stimulus. It is concluded that agility comes at a cost and that several trade-offs have to be considered when trying to increase organizational agility.

Characteristics of Command and Control in Response to
Emergencies and Disasters

The focus of this chapter by Trnka and Woltjer is the domain of command and control in emergency and disaster response operations. Response operations, as well as related command and control work, are characterized by loosely defined and shifting goals, versatile situations, time pressure, high stakes and the involvement of multiple organizations. The unique contexts and varying circumstances of response operations have an impact on how collaborative work and interactions among commanding personnel and organizations emerge. This emergence of response operations poses specific challenges and demands on commanding personnel and the organizations involved in this type of operation. The chapter identifies the main characteristics of different types of response operations and their implications for command and control. The focus is thereby on the need-based character of emergency and disaster response operations, as well as the need for adaptations of the responding organizations and their command and control structures. The article also describes key differences and commonalities between command and control in emergency and disaster response operations and military operations, and discusses their implications for joint operations.

Empirical Studies of Command and Control Centres at the Swedish Air Force

Svensson, Rencrantz, Marklund and Berggren describe how command and control environments are dynamic and complex settings with complicated technical systems where teams of operators interact to reach shared goals. The chapter presents two studies where evaluation techniques with dynamic measures were used. The studies sought to (a) develop evaluation methodologies for dynamic environments, (b) to validate the techniques and (c) to demonstrate their practicability in operational settings. The studies were conducted in air operations centres of the Swedish Air Force. Operators from the Swedish Air Force participated in both studies: a simulated peace support operation scenario in an operational setting, and operational activities as normal procedures. Data in terms of time series were collected by means of digital questionnaires, and items on aspects of mental workload, situation awareness, performance and vigilance were answered repeatedly. By means of factor analysis and structural equation modelling of data from the peace support study, a model which shows the causal relations between mental workload, individual performance and team performance was derived.

The findings give prominence to the repeated measurement technique and time series analysis. Dynamic factor analysis and structural equation modelling prove to be successful techniques for predicting changes of dynamic events. Individual predictions can be employed to diagnose and outline the operational status of groups or positions in command and control systems such as the command and control centres of the Swedish Air Force.

The Advance of a Valid and Reliable Tool for Assessing Shared Understanding

Berggren argues that team cognition is central to command and control where several people work together to accomplish a shared goal. A central research question within the command and control domain has been to assess the shared understanding of the common operational picture – to what degree do decision-makers share the same view and to what extent does that have an impact on their operational performance? Berggren presents the development of a tool for assessing shared understanding over six different experiments. The first experiment was conducted in a laboratory environment using students and non-specific questions. The second experiment used a military training facility with fighter pilots and the same non-specific questions. In the third experiment a microworld simulation was used with students rank-ordering the priorities of specific items. In the fourth experiment tank commanders rank-ordered the priorities of specific items. The fifth experiment was carried out in a military tank battalion training facility with commanders prioritizing self-generated items. The sixth study used trained participants prioritizing self-generated items in a controlled microworld experiment. As a result of these experiments, Berggren suggests a method that is quick to prepare, easy to use and easy to understand, and that captures shared understanding within a team of highly trained professionals.

Evaluating the Effectiveness of an Armoured Brigade Staff

In this chapter, Thunholm, Berggren and Wikberg present a study of the effectiveness of an armoured brigade headquarters (HQ) in three specific respects: (a) how the HQ staff is dimensioned in relation to its tasks, (b) how staff processes (i.e. planning, execution and coordination/decision) work and (c) how the HQ's Standard Operating Procedure and battle rhythm function, especially in the light of the HQ's organization and work processes. Designed as a survey study, the work is based on: (a) a military command team effectiveness instrument (CTEF 2.0); (b) measurement of workload according to Borg's scale; (c) subjective quality assessments of the brigade HQ's orders and reports; and (d) verification that the brigade HQ follows its Standard Operating Procedure. Fifty-four staff members of an armoured brigade HQ participated, facing the challenges of a peace support/ peacekeeping operation exercise.

Organizational Effectiveness at the Kosovo Force Headquarters

Granåsen and Marklund present the work performed by NATO RTO HFM-163 towards improving the organizational effectiveness of coalition operations, focusing on a case study of organizational effectiveness performed at NATO HQs in Kosovo. The aim was to validate a model of organizational effectiveness for a multinational coalition HQ developed within the HFM-163 project. According to this model, a number of input factors are involved, relating to people, structures, processes and culture, all affecting shared awareness, decision-making and information sharing in a multinational HQ.

The results show that the organizational effectiveness model developed by the HFM-163 research team is valid. A number of factors do have an effect on operative goals (i.e. information sharing, decision-making and shared awareness); some factors are of greater importance than others. For example, flexibility, leadership effectiveness, openness to diversity, trust and improvement orientation all have an impact on operational goals. Knowing which factors influence organizational effectiveness in a multinational HQ is a first important step in effectiveness improvement. The work of HFM-163 is a successful example of the benefits of a single research organization participating in a multinational research constellation such as that within the NATO RTO programme.

Agility in Command and Control – Functional Models of Cognition

Johansson discusses command and control agility in the light of functional models of cognition that are being used in the field of cognitive systems engineering. It is suggested that a command and control organization, just like any purposeful organism, must have or be able to execute a number of basic cognitive functions like goal setting, monitoring of such goals, regulation of action and so forth. In traditional and current command and control organizations and systems, such functions are bound to specific structures. In order to be command and control agile, the command and control organization/system must be able to move these functions across structures. In this context, Hollnagel's extended control model is used as an example of how a functional model of a cognitive system can be placed in a military context in order to illustrate agile command and control. It is suggested that context as well as the interaction between the antagonists and surrounding sources of power in the situation are important determinants for the degree of agility that is demanded in a specific situation. The agile command and control organization must be able to move between different states of stability and allocate and distribute their functions to fit evolving situations in order to survive.

Chapter 2
Analysing Tactical Cognitive Systems: Theories, Models and Methods

A. Norlander

Introduction

Complex dynamic processes and operations can be characterized as high-risk activities, where human team members and artefacts perform tasks together that require almost extreme mobility, efficiency, agility and endurance. Emergency management, air traffic control and military operations are all examples of missions where performance heavily – and increasingly – relies on distributed systems including numerous (separated) team players, who are 'forced' to coordinate their actions to attain high safety and effectiveness (without risking excessive resource depletion). In the future, commanders and operators will, to a greater extent, execute missions with operational and system characteristics that are dynamic and non-linear. This implies that seemingly 'small' actions or decisions may have serious and/or irreversible consequences for a mission as a whole. At the same time, the 'art' and practice of command and control, that is, tactics, techniques, procedures and training, to mention a few examples, constantly and concurrently need to strive for perfection. However, as Rochlin (1997) and others have observed, the specific skills and properties that systems, managers and operators indeed have to possess in order to yield optimal mission performance in such critical and uncertain situations are not easily identified. Consequently, skills and properties may be difficult to improve.

It is possible to draw several parallels with other work domains and research areas to uncover potential vulnerabilities inherent in multiparty, high-risk activities. In this regard, areas of particular interest are, for example, commercial aviation and air traffic control (Smith et al. 1997); process control, management and systems theory (Forrester 1961; Senge 1990; Sheridan 1997); dynamic, distributed decision-making (Brehmer 1991, 1992; Brehmer and Allard 1991; Rasmussen et al. 1991); and naturalistic decision-making (Zsambok and Klein 1997).

In these types of activities, decisions and actions are never isolated events. Rather, they occur in the context(s) of, for example, stress (and its effects), uncertain evidence, ambiguous information, time pressure and time delays, or high physical and mental workload. Other important factors may be conflicting goals (that is, organizational and social aspects), minor actions that may trigger, as it were, large consequences, or simply highly dynamic, sometimes even chaotic, environments.

To address complex high-risk activities, we integrated well-established scientific disciplines into a pioneering research direction called *action control theory* (ACT), a framework specifically composed to facilitate empirically based conceptual modelling of dynamic, complex tactical systems and processes, as well as their states and state transitions. The resulting models are to be used for complex, multi-level human–machine systems design in the military, aviation and emergency response domains.

The Action Control Theory Framework

Action control theory can be argued to be a composite theoretical structure deriving its primary constituents from advances in four areas: (a) cognitive systems engineering (CSE), (b) systems theory, control theory and cybernetics, (c) decision-making in complex systems control and mission command, and (d) psychophysiology.

These four research areas (constituting ACT) have until now developed as separate paths; however, the time has come to investigate what they might offer when combined and implemented in an integrated, cohesive and coordinated manner. Flach and Kuperman (1998) conclude that it is essential to develop a unified, proactive, CSE-based approach in research and systems design for future warfare environments. Norlander (2010) describes the power and utility of integrated research approaches that are built on solid classical and innovative theoretical work. However, Norlander also emphasizes the need for support from advanced experimental and measurement methods and data analysis techniques. Applying theory and analysis in concert enables the development of comprehensive yet simple and robust conceptual and specific models of systems, tasks and missions.

Theoretical Constituent I: Cognitive Systems Engineering

The field of cognitive systems engineering has steadily grown since the first significant contributions were published in the 1980s by Rasmussen (1983, 1986), who introduced the concept of skill-, rule- and knowledge-based behaviour for the modelling of different levels of human performance. A decade later, Endsley (1995) developed a comprehensive theory of individual operator, commander and team situation awareness in dynamic systems. Danielsson and Ohlsson (1996) studied information needs and information quality in emergency management decision-making, a work which also applies to the military context. Woods and Roth (1988) made a comprehensive review of the CSE domain. Hollnagel and Woods (1983) made a significant contribution to this field through their definition of a cognitive system (CS) as a man–machine system (MMS) whose behaviour is goal-oriented, based on symbol manipulation and employs heuristic knowledge of its surrounding environment for guidance. A cognitive system operates by using knowledge about itself and a given environment to plan and modify its actions based on precisely that knowledge (Rasmussen et al. 1994). As for complex systems, such knowledge is indisputable. For example, in command and control tasks in military missions a multitude of sensor systems, communication systems, training programmes, personnel and procedures are all elements of a 'wider' (total) operational system (Rencrantz et al. 2006). The total operational capability is built from a set of capability elements: *doctrine, organization, training, material, leadership, personnel, facilities* and *interoperability* (abbreviated as DOTMLPFI).

Looking upon this system as a cognitive system permits the integration of all capability elements into an adaptive distributed system that can achieve a mission safely and efficiently. The use of CSE to model, analyse and describe such systems performing hazardous, real-time, high-stakes activities is effective, given that operators and analysts alike have sufficient understanding of the interdependencies, linkages between other research areas and the CSE field (Norlander 2009).

Theoretical Constituent II:
Dynamic Systems Theory, Control Theory and Cybernetics

The term dynamic system refers to an object driven by external input signals $u(t)$ for every value of time t which, as a response, produces a set of output signals $y(t)$ for every t. Ashby (1956) and Brehmer (1992), among others, have shown that most complex systems have real-time, dynamic properties. The system output at a given time not only depends on the input value at that specific moment, but also on earlier input values. A good regulator of a system also has to implement a model of the system that can be (that is to be) controlled. Put somewhat differently, Ashby's law of requisite variety (Ashby 1956) states that the variety of a controller (also called regulator) of a dynamic system has to be equal to, or greater than, the variety of the system itself.

An approach based on control theory and dynamic systems can facilitate structuring and understanding of command and control problems. The mathematical stringency and formalism of control theory makes it possible to describe and treat technical, organizational, economic and biological dynamic systems in basically the same manner: as processes or clusters of processes, with a built-in, or external, control system. Further, concepts of control theory can be used as metaphors in research on decision-making, especially in complex, dynamic contexts where many operators, systems and other entities are active simultaneously. The fact that decision-making regulates command and control processes (Orhaug 1995) heavily supports a control theory approach. The traditional hierarchical command structures of military forces and emergency response organizations are strongly coupled to both centralized and distributed decision-making principles (Brehmer 1988).

However, the areas of control theory and decision theory have evolved considerably since the mid 1990s. Research by Alberts (2011) shows that in extraordinarily complex, uncertain and challenging endeavours, mission performance improves significantly when the command and control function decentralizes decision rights and improves information availability throughout the force, making the organization more resilient, adaptive and agile. Annett (1997) uses control theory to investigate team skills, which indicates the usefulness of the control theory framework for analysis and evaluation of command and control in tactical operations. It is to be observed that four fundamental requirements must be met (Conant and Ashby 1970; Glad and Ljung 1989; Brehmer 1992) if control theory is to be used in the analysis and synthesis of dynamic systems. First, the system must have a clear mission related to a goal (the goal condition). Second, it must be possible to ascertain the state of the system through observation and measurement (the observability condition). Third, it must be possible to influence and modify the state of the system (the controllability condition). Lastly, the regulator controlling the system is dependent on the existence of an internal model of the system (the model condition).

Controlling Joint Systems and Processes

The combined view of control theory in technical as well in behavioural domains is crucial for success in ACT-based research. When a function is implemented at one level of abstraction, represented at a second level of abstraction and controlled at a third level of abstraction, the requirements for timely and complete information varies accordingly. On the other hand, it is not important whether a function or mission is carried out by an operator or by an automated system under higher-order supervision. Operators and supervisory controllers still need to maintain adequate situation understanding or situation awareness. If reliable and timely observation and measurement of a system output is unfeasible and situation understanding cannot be based on the information supplied by the system, it must be based on current process knowledge and an understanding of a given situation. Operators and controllers must thus compensate using accurate predictions of system performance. Such prediction ability is based on the axiom that a cognitive system must be able to think ahead in time and also anticipate the dynamics of the process. To accomplish this goal, a cognitive system must solely rely on exact model knowledge of the influence of the system's input on the system output. This is usually referred to as open-loop control. This type of control can be a cumbersome, arduous task, especially when a system environment and mission context is dynamic and the system process is unstable and non-linear. Sometimes, small changes or state transitions in a process may generate disproportionate, unpredictable, even chaotic system behaviour. In some cases, such disturbances can be measured, making it possible to eliminate the influence of the disturbances by using feed-forward control. It is to be observed, however, that this requires extremely good system knowledge of the process that is to be controlled. Feed-forward control is also sensitive to variability in system dynamics.

The main advantage of feed-forward control is the possibility of counteracting the effects of disturbances before they are visible as undesired deviations from the reference. Control theory has proven that although feed-forward control can be considered the perfect mode of control, it is often only achievable for a limited time due to model errors caused by, among other things, the time constants of a process. However, if the system output can be used to determine the system state, there is only a limited need for detailed knowledge of system dynamics, and feedback control can be maintained. The necessary adjustments and updates of the controller's internal system model can be made by constantly measuring the deviation of the system output from the reference value. The joint cognitive system is a learning system, thus unstable without feedback. Feedback is needed to correct deviations and compensate for the incompleteness and inadequacy of the internal system model. Reason (1997) emphasizes the importance of this balance between feedback (reactive or compensatory) control and feed-forward (proactive or anticipatory) control. The concept of the feedback–feed-forward control balance is crucial if the cognitive system is to achieve optimal performance in a tactical mission.

Theoretical Constituent III: Dynamic Decision-making in Complex Systems Control and Mission Command

Brehmer (1992) suggests control theory as a framework for research in distributed, dynamic decision-making. The conventional view of decision-making, supported by normative theories, 'reduces' decision-making to the selection of appropriate action(s) from a closed, predefined action set and to the resolution of conflicting choices. As a consequence, the analysis of decision tasks focuses on the generation of alternatives and the evaluation of these alternatives, as in, for example, multi-attribute utility (MAU) analysis (Kleindorfer et al. 1993). Research in dynamic decision-making has been based on analysis of several applied scenarios, for example military decision-making, operator tasks in industrial processes, emergency management and intensive care (Brehmer 1988, 1992). Two things were clarified in these analyses. First, the decision-making was never the primary task. It was always directed towards some goal. Second, the dynamic character of the assigned tasks became apparent in the study of the applied contexts. These results are consistent with earlier descriptions of dynamic decision-making (DDM) by Edwards (1962), Rapoport (1975) and Hogarth (1981). The early work on DDM was integrated by Brehmer (1992) with his own research on decision-making in time-critical situations, and he formulated a set of common DDM characteristics, described as follows. A series of decisions is required to reach a specific goal; to achieve and maintain control is a continuous activity requiring many decisions, each of which can be understood only in the context of the other decisions. Decisions are mutually dependent. Later decisions are constrained by earlier decisions and, in turn, constrain those that come thereafter. The state of a specific decision problem changes, both autonomously and as a consequence of the decision-maker's actions. Decisions have to be made in real time; this finding has several significant implications and is elaborated upon in the next section.

Real-time properties of dynamic decision-making cause certain problems. Initially, decision-makers are not free to make decisions when they feel ready to do so. Instead, the mission environment requires decisions, and a decision-maker – ready or not – has to make these decisions more or less on demand, something which causes stress in dynamic decision-making tasks. In order to cope with this stress, decision-makers have to develop strategies for controlling assigned dynamic tasks and for keeping their own workload at an acceptable level. Additionally, both the system that is to be controlled and the procedures and resources the decision-maker employs to control the system have to be seen and treated as processes. Dynamic decision-making tasks can therefore be characterized as finding a way to use one process to control another process. Lastly, the different time scales involved in dynamic decision-making tasks have to be monitored and taken into consideration. In most situations, the active agents in a dynamic system, such as the directly involved operators and their closest commander or squad leader, operate in a time scale of seconds to minutes. Their commanders and their command and control systems operate in time scales of hours to days. An application of this approach in studies of distributed decision-making in dynamic environments, such as fire-fighting and rescue missions, is described by Brehmer and Svenmarck (1995).

Naturalistic Approaches to Decision-making

Zachary and Ryder (1997) review decision-making research during the last four decades and elaborate a recent paradigm shift in decision theory. The shift develops from analytic, normative decision-making procedures (described in Kleindorfer et al. 1993) to naturalistic decision-making (see Klein 1993a, 1993b; Klein and Woods 1993; Zsambok and Klein 1997). Naturalistic decision-making applies to several dynamic and potentially dangerous activity areas such as military missions, air traffic control, fire-fighting, emergency response and medical care, which all share the central characteristics of the naturalistic decision-making paradigm. First and foremost, human decision-making should be studied in its natural context. Then, the task at hand and the operational situation is critical for successful framing of a decision problem. Consequently, actions and decisions are highly interrelated. Experts apply their experience and knowledge non-analytically by identifying and effecting the most appropriate action in an intuitive manner.

Cannon-Bowers et al. (1996) review, comment on and relate naturalistic decision-making to extensive research on distributed and dynamic decision-making (as described above). Their conclusion is that naturalistic decision-making offers a practical and empirically well-founded research approach to overcome the limitations of the notions of the classic normative research paradigm in decision-making. A fundamental element of naturalistic decision-making, the recognition-primed decision model, is presented in detail in Klein (1993a) and applied to complex command and control environments in, for example, Kaempf et al. (1996).

Tactical Team Decision-making

Tactical decision-making teams in modern warfare environments face situations characterized by rapidly unfolding events, multiple concurrent hypotheses of future events and required decisions, high information ambiguity, severe time pressure and risks of serious consequences of error and failure (Cannon-Bowers et al. 1995). There are also instances when large geographical distances or other forms of distributed environments in which the teams operate impose additional difficulties (Brehmer 1991). To adapt to these situations, team members must coordinate their actions so that they can gather, process, integrate and communicate information in a timely and effective manner (Svensson et al. 2006). This is particularly relevant for complex adaptive systems, where it is difficult to assess performance with a single correct answer or in situations where several individual decision-makers must interact as a team.

Theoretical Constituent IV: Psychophysiology

Within joint cognitive systems performing complex, high-risk military and emergency response missions, there is a fundamental and deep connection between a human operator's physiological stress response, on the one hand, and discrepancies between expectations and experiences, on the other hand. The stress response indicates a homeostatic imbalance (Levine and Ursin 1991); the concept of model error (from control theory) can be applied once again. A stress response also mobilizes physiological resources to improve performance, something which in itself may be regarded as a positive and desirable warning response. The cognitive activation theory of stress (CATS) describes phases of stress responses as alarms occurring within complex adaptive cognitive systems with feedback and feed-forward control loops – no less, but no more, complicated than any other of the body's self-regulated systems (Eriksen et al. 1999). The time dimension of stress responses must, however, be accounted for very carefully.

Models Derived From Action Control Theory

The point of departure in our ACT-based systems modelling endeavour is the definition of a so-called *tactical joint cognitive system* (TJCS). In practice, a TJCS is a system to which the mission is assigned, to which the assets necessary for mission engagement and sustainment are allocated and to which tactical command of the mission is assigned. It is given the responsibility of accomplishing the mission and is provided the authority, responsibility and resources needed for performing the mission successfully.

Worm (2002) describes the TJCS as an aggregate of at least one – but often several – instances of each of the following subsystem classes: (a) *mission systems*, with the aim of engaging, deploying and informing, for example vehicles and other platforms, effects systems (that is, weapons or other systems for direct or indirect influence), intelligence acquisition systems, communication systems, sensors and other reconnaissance systems, along with all mission-essential system operators; (b) *command-and-control systems*, including certain mission system components, dedicated technological systems, decision support functions, an information exchange and command architecture, higher-level doctrine and directly involved decision-makers; (c) *sustainment and protection systems*, comprising logistic functions, staff functions, various organizational structures, protection and life support systems, doctrine, tactics and procedures, staff and mission training and various kinds of service support; and (d) *tactical teams*, composed of and defined according to Salas et al. (1992) as two or more people who interact, dynamically, interdependently and adaptively toward a common and valued goal/objective/ mission, who have been assigned specific roles or functions to perform, and who have a limited lifespan of membership. The TJCS concept is depicted in Figure 2.1.

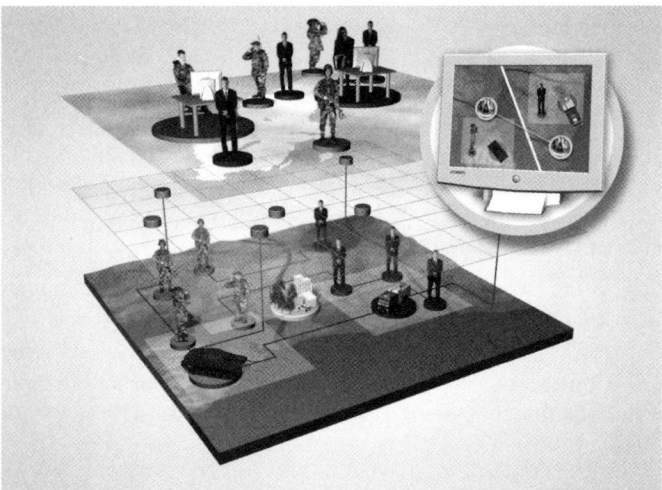

Figure 2.1   The tactical joint cognitive system. Mission systems, command and control systems, sustainment and protection systems and tactical teams interact dynamically and interdependently towards mission accomplishment

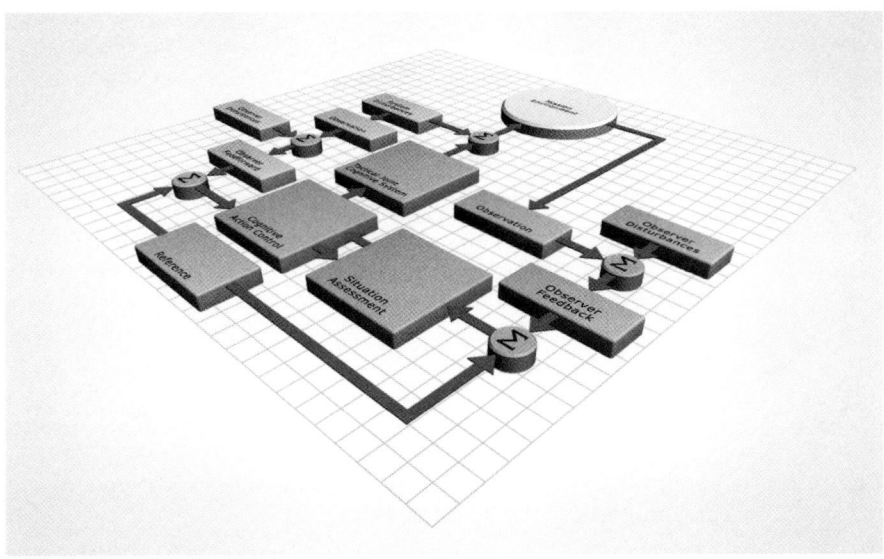

Figure 2.2   The tactical action control model (TACOM). Its principal components are connected through flows of matter, energy and information

There are other important characteristics of a team in a TJCS, one being how a mission in itself affects performance. Serfaty and Entin (1997) draw the following conclusions concerning the properties and abilities of teams successfully performing tactical, hazardous operations. To begin with, the team structure adapts to changes in the task environment. This secures competence, skill, performance and effectiveness. The team maintains open and flexible communication lines. This is especially important in situations where so-called lower levels in a command hierarchy have access to critical information that is not available to higher command levels. Team members are extremely sensitive to the workload and performance of other members in high-tempo/high-stakes situations.

Tactical Action Control Models

We then turn our attention to the tactical action control model (TACOM, Worm 2000a), as illustrated in Figure 2.2. The four principal components of the TACOM are the mission environment, the tactical joint cognitive system, the situation assessment function and the cognitive action control function, derived primarily from Brehmer (1988, 1992), Klein (1993a, 1993b) and Worm (1998c, 2000b). There are relationships between these components, originally described by Miller (1978), one of the founders of *living systems theory* (LST).

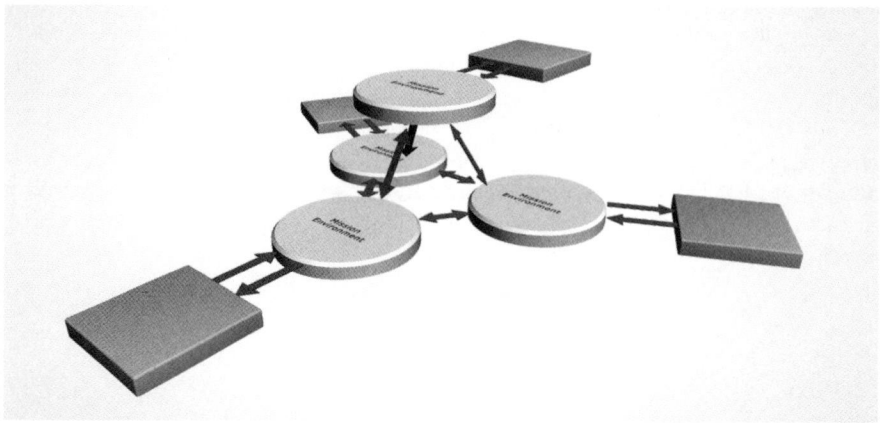

Figure 2.3   A simplified example of a multi-level mission execution and control model (MULTI-MECOM)

Living systems theory offers a means for analysing the structure, function and processes of organizations and finding shortcomings that reduce a system's effectiveness in achieving its objectives. These subsystems are related to each other by the processing and exchange of matter, energy and information. In the general case, these relations are often non-linear, sometimes non-deterministic or, in unstable or conflicting cases, even chaotic.

Mission Execution and Control Models

The next step is to integrate these concepts into what we call a *mission execution and control model* (MECOM). The MECOM combines several command and control strategies and is therefore an agile system, capable of successfully effecting, coping with, and/or exploiting changes in the surrounding mission environment (Alberts 2011). It consists of one or several TACOMs extended with additional control functions and components to handle system disturbances, model error and to allow an adaptive, balanced mix of feed-forward and feedback control. The MECOM structure is presented in Figure 2.3.

The MECOM aggregate is derived from central concepts and principles of the cognitive systems engineering field, where cognition and control are always embedded in a context. The model assumes adaptability and agility to successfully effect, cope with, and/or exploit changes in the surrounding mission environment. The context includes demands and resources, tasks, goals, organization, decision rights, information richness, social and physical factors and situation dynamics. When modelling cognitive processes, such as command, control and intelligence processes, one must account for how cognition depends on the overall context rather than on the input alone. Procedural prototype control models assume a characteristic sequence of actions, whose ordering is determined by the control prototype (Hollnagel 1998). Contextual control models, however, focus on how the choice of next action is determined mainly by the current context of the mission (or purpose). Contextual control models describe action sequences as constructed rather than previously defined. The choice of action is controlled by the context, and actions can be both reactive and proactive. Contextual control models make a distinction between competence and control, in that competence – or in other words, capability – describes what the operator and commander is able to do, and control describes how he achieves it.

Method

In earlier publications (Worm 1998b, 1999a, 1999b) we have reported on the progress of the project Tactical Real-time Interaction in Distributed Environments (TRIDENT), aimed at developing a coherent, straightforward 'package' of methods and techniques for man–machine systems analysis in the setting of tactical mission scenarios. The components of TRIDENT are described in Table 2.1.

Table 2.1   The components of the TRIDENT methods and techniques package

Method/Tool/Technique	Reference/s
Using the ACT framework for conceptual modelling of dynamic, complex adaptive tactical systems and processes, of their states and state transitions	Worm (2000a)
Identification of mission and unit state variables and of action control and decision-making mechanisms for process regulation	Worm (1998a, 1998b)
Mission efficiency analysis (of fully manned and equipped units executing full-scale tactical missions in an authentic environment	Worm et al. (1998); Worm (1999a)
Measuring information distribution and communication effectiveness	Worm (1998b)
Measuring workload by means of the NASA task load index (NASA-TLX)	Hart and Staveland (1988)
Assessing team member psychosocial mood by means of the mood adjective checklist (MACL)	Sjöberg et al. (1979)
Assessing situation awareness as a function of mission-critical information complexity	Svensson et al. (1993); Endsley (1995)
Measuring level and mode of cognitive, context-dependent control of the team members and identifying what control strategies were utilized by the team and team members	Hollnagel (1998)
Applying reliability and error analysis methods for investigating failure causes both in retrospect and for prediction	Hollnagel (1998)
Validating identified constructs and measuring their influence using advanced data analytic procedures	Svensson et al. (2006)

Implementing our ideas for tactical mission analysis has proven to be both cost-effective and applicable in a multitude of high-risk, stressful and cognitively complex situations and environments. Using the TRIDENT concepts for analysis and evaluation of aggregated system levels has so far been rewarding, with high acceptance by subjects such as trained and skilled professionals performing their daily tasks in their regular work environment. Numerous battle management and emergency response studies have been carried out in which we have tested, refined and augmented the modelling, measurement, data collection and analysis concepts described above. However, we have also experienced some critique. It is occasionally claimed that the reliability and validity of subjective workload ratings are insufficient. For that reason, we incorporated a measure of workload and stress which is commonly accepted in the scientific community, namely hormonal response measures. Settling on this decision, we were influenced by the results of Svensson et al. (1993), who studied workload and performance in military aviation; Zeier (1994), who analysed workload and stress reactions in air traffic controllers; and Holmboe et al. (1975), who examined military personnel performing exhausting battle training.

We designed a study in order to elucidate to what extent hormonal physiological stress indications indeed are linked to the rating, observation and data collection methods normally used in TRIDENT to assess workload and tactical performance. The study was originally described in Worm (2000a).

Participants

The subjects were officers and conscripts, organized in a small, agile distributed battalion command staff, consisting of one forward command post, designated L1, and one tactical operations centre, designated L3. L1 was in operational command, handling all operational battalion-level decisions, but was also responsible for action execution in the second-to-minute time perspective. L1 comprised a tactical command team of six operators, four of whom were professional military officers: one battalion commander (CDR), one operations officer (OPS), one intelligence officer (INT) and one fire/weapons coordination officer (WEAP). The team also included two conscript staff assistants/signal specialists.

L3 handled all services not covered by L1, such as combat support services, long-term mission planning and intelligence activities and provided backup and relief to the tactical command team in L1 when necessary. The L3 tactical operations team consisted of 10 officers and four soldiers in total. It included one tactical command team, similar to the forward-deployed L1 team, and one tactical operations team: one quartermaster (QMR), one logistics officer (LOG), one C3I systems officer (COMMS), one air defence officer (AD), one technical officer (TECHS) and one combat engineering officer (ENG) with expertise in mine clearance, mine laying, combat bridging and other engineering support. The four L3 conscripts were staff assistants/signal specialists.

The officers were between 27 and 38 years of age, with a minimum of six years of service after commission. The officers formed a hardened team, with extensive professional experience, ranging from two to ten years of practice in their respective current battalion staff position from various national and international missions. The conscripts were in their early 20s, had finished basic soldier training and were in the final phase of their specialist training for their intended wartime assignments.

Material

The study was carried out at a command post-training facility (CPTF) designed for training two fully manned battalion staffs. The system was dimensioned for simulating two battalion-sized ground warfare units engaging an enemy force of comparable capacity. Each unit could be assigned joint or independent missions in different areas of operations in a larger-scale brigade or division scenario. In the CPTF, all units are represented as simulated, virtual units. Exercise leaders of each unit undergoing training are situated in the exercise control centre, controlling the actions of all their subordinated units. Unit manoeuvring is determined by pre-programmed system parameters, updated in real time if necessary. The simulation system monitors depletion and replenishment of resources and supplies, and updates resource records available to the trainees and the exercise control function. When units manoeuvre within a specific engagement distance, the simulation simply pauses and the exercise controllers determine the outcome of the engagement. Parametric simulation models then yield the distribution of casualties and destroyed systems.

Procedure

The context of the study was a five-day brigade-level simulated ground warfare scenario. This global scenario continued through the whole study and was composed of six consecutive battalion-level engagements. Each engagement constituted one complete battalion combat scenario, divided into three phases: a) manoeuvring to the deployment zone and advancement to the assembly area, b) advancement to final assault position and enemy engagement and c) reassembly after engagement and preparing for the next mission as stated in the brigade operations orders.

Losses and depleted resources after one battalion combat scenario were carried into the next scenario or experimental session, unless refuelling and restoration of ammunition and other supplies were (or could be) foreseen and prepared by the battalion commander and staff. The first two sessions were used for acclimatization and additional training, to eliminate training effects and to ensure individual performance consistency through the following four sessions. During the four subsequent experimental sessions, each phase of the scenario contained one testing juncture. For every testing juncture, a 'time-out' was announced at which saliva samples were collected in Sarstedt's salivette devices (individually marked test tubes containing a small sterile cotton swab). A short questionnaire (three open questions and three rating questions) on a subject's level of situational control regarding available time, space and resources was also administered during each testing juncture. The time-out only lasted for as long as was needed for everyone to saturate the cotton swab and to put it back into the saliva test tube (approximately three minutes). During this time period, subjects had time to answer the short questionnaire.

After every completed experimental session a longer, more comprehensive, questionnaire was administered (totalling 69 rating questions), by which all subjects individually rated their own mental and physical workload, psychosocial mood, situation awareness and battle command information complexity during the session.

We collected a total of 77 saliva samples, 11 from each one of seven key-position staff members (CDR/L1, OPS/L1, OPS/L3, INT/L3, WEAP/L1, FIRES/L3 and QMR/L3). The seven subjects were selected based on an assessment of which team roles were the most likely to experience high levels of cognitive stress in high-intensity ground warfare missions. They were selected by means of their job requirements, expert consultation and a predictive cognitive reliability and error analysis. The decision not to collect saliva samples from all subjects was due to laboratory cost considerations. However, we administered the control level questionnaires to all subjects. After every experimental session we administered the long questionnaires to all 20 subjects, on six occasions in total. The test tubes were stored at -20°C during transport to the analysis laboratory at the Occupational and Environmental Medicine Division, Linköping University, Faculty of Health Sciences. Due to personal integrity and research ethics, all questionnaires and observation protocols were codified and all linkage to the saliva samples and the subjects was made by an alphanumerical reference code only.

Results

The individual catecholamine responses in the third and fourth sessions are shown in Figure 2.4. From this we found that the battalion commander (CDR/L1) reacted in connection with phase 1 in every session, while the operations officer (OPS/L1) tended to react more in connection with phase 2. The fire/weapons coordinator (WEAP/L1) showed a considerably higher and more stable catecholamine response, although peaking in the same phase as CDR/L1. However, as can be seen in Figure 2.5, from the control level ratings we found that the subjects individually, as well as a team, rated their control level higher than their hormonal response indicated, until they encountered a difficult situation in phase 2 in the fourth session.

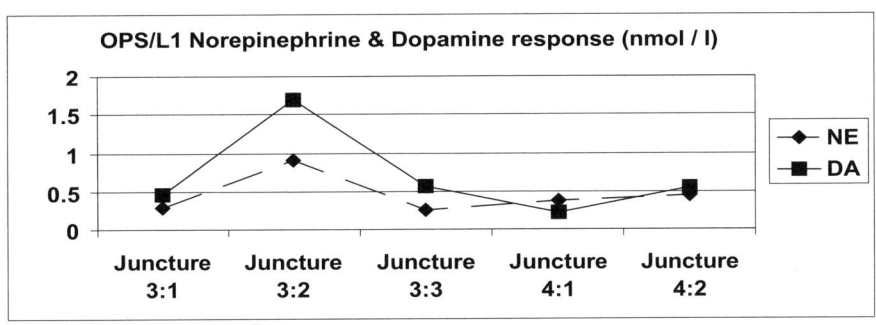

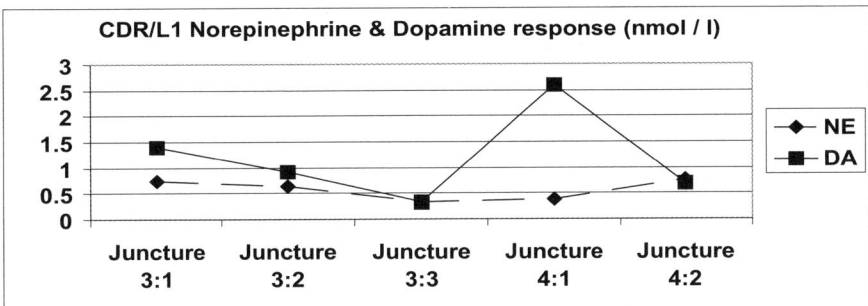

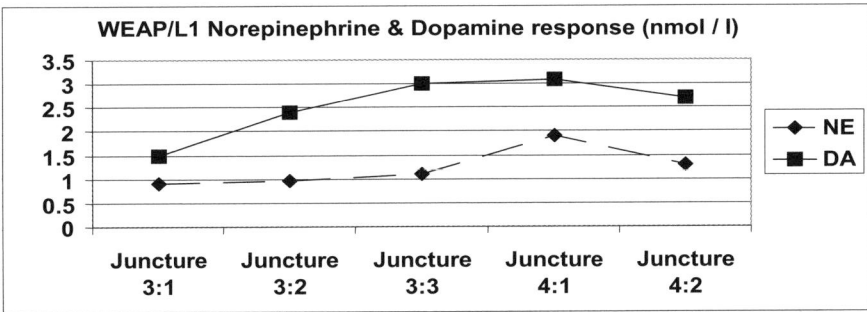

Figure 2.4   Individual catecholamine response (nmol/l) in team L1 (CDR, OPS and WEAP)

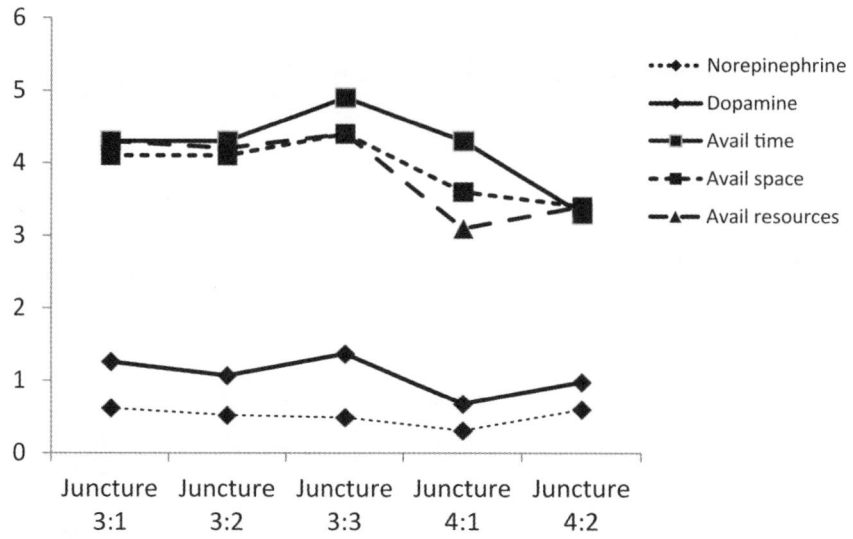

Figure 2.5   Aggregated catecholamine levels (nmol/l) vs rated level of control (rating 0 to 7) in team L1 (CDR, OPS and WEAP)

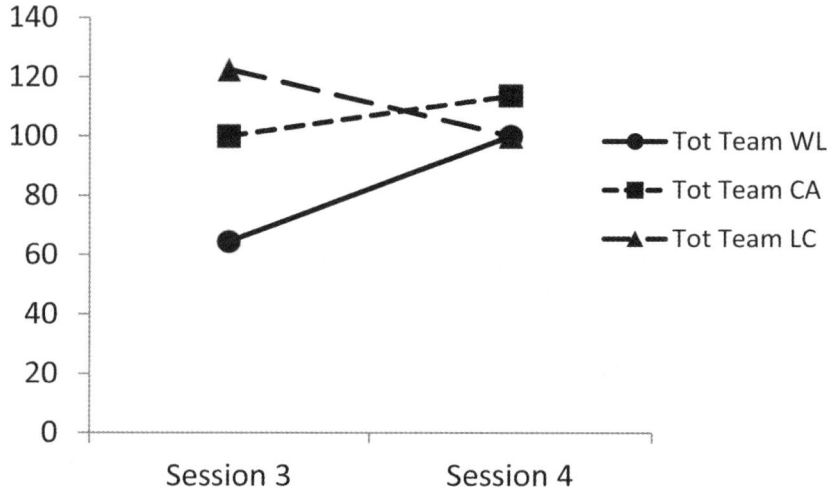

Figure 2.6   Aggregated catecholamine levels (CA) vs rated level of control (LC) vs rated workload (WL)

When team-wise aggregated NASA-TLX workload ratings were considered (as shown in Figure 2.6), we found a positive relationship between self-rated workload and catecholamine response, and a negative relationship between the aforementioned factors and self-rated level of control.

Figure 2.6 shows values from team L1 (CDR, OPS and WEAP); the data has been scaled to a nominal value of 100.

Discussion

Our results suggest three potentially significant mechanisms influencing how a team is able to execute mission control, which consequently also influences mission efficiency. First, the influence of stress on individual and team performance is linked to time-dependent filtering functions like defence and coping mechanisms according to the cognitive *activation theory of stress* (Levine and Ursin 1991; Eriksen et al. 1999). Second, team performance depends on individual mission task requirements (Worm 2000a). Third, overall mission performance critically depends on an adaptive and agile balance between feed-forward and feedback in action control according to the action control theory (Worm 2000a).

Implementing our ideas in tactical mission analysis in potentially dangerous, stressful and cognitively complex environments was indeed effective and very rewarding. Using the ACT/TRIDENT approach facilitated several activities necessary to perform advanced systems engineering for mission-critical applications: ACT/TRIDENT provides the means to identify the limiting factors of a specific individual, unit, system, procedure or mission. ACT aids the assessment of the magnitude of influence of these limiting factors on overall tactical performance. Furthermore, this analysis and assessment approach makes it quite straightforward to generate and implement measures to support and improve insufficient capabilities and contribute to successful accomplishment of future missions. The TRIDENT method package offers methodological support to analysis, evaluation and development of future integrated mission support systems. It also supports improvement of training programmes for tactical decision-making and mission management.

Concluding Remarks

The life-threatening environment in which military and crisis response units operate stresses the need for clear-cut, unambiguous principles, concepts and structures for command and control, and high-performance integrated command and control systems working in concert with strategic, operational and tactical doctrine.

One prerequisite for success in future military and crisis response missions is support from highly capable command, control, communications and intelligence (C3I), enabling every commander and operator to develop a comprehensive and detailed system insight and situation understanding, leading to safe and efficient mission accomplishment. The potentials of high-capacity information processing and real-time interaction in a distributed, dynamic mission environment need to be fully exploited.

We have worked towards building a foundation for analysis and evaluation of high-stakes, life-threatening tactical missions in various work contexts. Based on the analysis of the study reported in this chapter and on extensive work performed by others, we contend that studying individuals is an effective, reliable and valid way to probe the function and efficiency of an organization performing complex tasks in ever-changing mission environments.

References

Alberts, D.S. (2011). *The Agility Advantage: A Survival Guide for Complex Enterprises and Endeavors*. Washington, DC: US DoD Command and Control Research Program.

Annett, J. (1997). Analysing team skills. In R. Flin, E. Salas, M. Strub and L. Martin (eds), *Decision-making Under Stress: Emerging Themes and Applications*. Aldershot: Ashgate, 315–25.

Ashby, W.R. (1956). *An Introduction to Cybernetics*. London: Chapman & Hall.

Brehmer, B. (1988). Organization of decision-making in complex systems. In L.P. Goodstein, H.B. Andersen and S.E. Olesen (eds), *Tasks, Errors, and Mental Models*. London: Taylor & Francis.

Brehmer, B. (1991). Time scales, distributed decision-making, and modern information technology. In J. Rasmussen, B. Brehmer and J. Leplat (eds), *Distributed Decision-making: Cognitive Models for Cooperative Work*. Chichester: Wiley.

Brehmer, B. (1992). Dynamic decision-making: Human control of complex systems. *Acta Psychologica*, 81, 211–41.

Brehmer, B. and Allard, R. (1991). Real-time dynamic decision-making: The effects of task complexity and feedback delays. In J. Rasmussen, B. Brehmer and J. Leplat (eds), *Distributed Decision-making: Cognitive Models for Cooperative Work*. Chichester: Wiley.

Brehmer, B. and Svenmarck, P. (1995). Distributed decision-making in dynamic environments: Time scales and architectures of decision-making. In J.P. Caverni, M. Bar-Hillel, F.H. Barron and H. Jungermann (eds), *Contributions to Decision-making I*. Amsterdam: Elsevier Science B.V.

Cannon-Bowers, J.A., Salas, E. and Pruitt, J.S. (1996). Establishing the boundaries of a paradigm for decision-making research. *Human Factors*, 38, 193–205.

Cannon-Bowers, J.A., Tannenbaum, S.I., Salas, E. and Volpe, C.E. (1995). Defining team competencies and establishing team training requirements. In R. Guzzo and E. Salas (eds), *Team Effectiveness and Decision-making in Organizations*. San Francisco, CA: Jossey Bass, 333–80.

Conant, R.C. and Ashby, W.R. (1970). Every good regulator of a system must be a model of that system. *International Journal of System Science*, 1, 89–97.

Danielsson, M. and Ohlsson, K. (1996). Models of decision-making in emergency management. *Proceedings of the 1st International Conference on Engineering Psychology and Cognitive Ergonomics*, Stratford-upon-Avon, 23–5 October 1996. Cranfield: Cranfield University.

Edwards, W. (1962). Dynamic decision theory and probabilistic information processing. *Human Factors*, 4, 59–73.

Endsley, M.R. (1995). Towards a theory for situation awareness in dynamic systems. *Human Factors*, 37, 32–64.

Eriksen, H.R., Olff, M., Murison, R. and Ursin, H. (1999). The time dimension in stress responses: Relevance for survival and health. *Psychiatry Research*, 85, 39–50.

Flach, J.M. and Kuperman, G. (1998). *Victory by Design: War, Information, and Cognitive Systems Engineering* (Report No. AFRL–HE–WP–TR–1998–0074). Wright-Patterson AFB, OH: Air Force Research Laboratory, Crew System Interface Division.

Forrester, J.W. (1961). *Industrial Dynamics*. Portland, OR: Productivity Press.

Glad, T. and Ljung, L. (1989). *Reglerteknik. Grundläggande teori*. [Automatic Control. Basic Theory.] Lund: Studentlitteratur.

Hart, S.G. and Staveland, L.E. (1988). Development of a multi-dimensional workload rating scale: Results of empirical and theoretical research. In P.A. Hancock and N. Meshkati (eds), *Human Mental Workload*. Amsterdam: Elsevier Science B.V.

Hogarth, R.M. (1981). Beyond discrete biases: Functional and dysfunctional aspects of judgmental heuristics. *Psychological Bulletin*, 90, 197–317.

Hollnagel, E. (1998). *Cognitive Reliability and Error Analysis Method (CREAM)*. Amsterdam: Elsevier Science B.V.

Hollnagel, E. and Woods, D.D. (1983). Cognitive systems engineering: New wine in new bottles. *International Journal of Man–Machine Studies*, 18, 583–600.

Holmboe, J., Bell, H. and Norman, N. (1975). Urinary excretion of catecholamines and steroids in military cadets exposed to prolonged stress. *Försvarsmedicin*, 11, 183.

Kaempf, G.L., Klein, G.A., Thordsen, M.L. and Wolf, S. (1996). Decision-making in complex command and control environments. *Human Factors*, 38, 220–31.

Klein, G.A. (1993a). *Naturalistic Decision-making – Implications for Design*. State-of-the-Art Report. Dayton, OH: Crew Systems Ergonomics Information Analysis Center, Wright-Patterson Air Force Base.

Klein, G.A. (1993b). A recognition-primed decision (RPD) model of rapid decision-making. In G.A. Klein, J. Orasanu, R. Calderwood and C.E. Zsambok (eds), *Decision-making in Action: Models and Methods*. Norwood, NJ: Ablex.

Klein, G.A. and Woods, D.D. (1993). Conclusions: Decision-making in action. In G.A. Klein, J. Orasanu, R. Calderwood and C.E. Zsambok (eds), *Decision-making in Action: Models and Methods*. Norwood, NJ: Ablex.

Kleindorfer, P.R., Kunhreuther, H.C. and Schoemaker, P.J. (1993). *Decision Sciences. An Integrative Perspective*. Cambridge: Cambridge University Press.

Levine, S. and Ursin, H. (1991). What is stress? In M.R. Brown, G.F. Koob and C. Rivier (eds), *Stress – Neurobiology and Neuroendocrinology*. New York: Marcel Dekker, 3–21.

Miller, J.G. (1978). *Living Systems*. New York: McGraw-Hill.

Norlander, A. (2009). Representation and control of complex joint human–machine systems: An information and sense making perspective. In *Proceedings of the American Society of Naval Engineers Human Systems Integration Symposium 2009*. Alexandria, VA: The American Society of Naval Engineers.

Norlander, A. (2010). Analysis of tactical missions: Integrating systems theory, cognitive systems engineering and psychophysiology. In *Proceedings of the Human Factors and Ergonomics Society 54th Annual Meeting*. Santa Monica, CA: The Human Factors Society.

Orhaug, T. (1995). *Ledningsvetenskap – En diskussion av beskrivningsmässiga och teoretiska problem inom ledningsområdet*. [Science of command and control – A discussion of descriptive and theoretical problems within the domain of command and control.] Stockholm: The Swedish National Defence College.

Rapoport, A. (1975). Research paradigms for the study of dynamic decision behavior. In D. Wendt and C. Vlek (eds), *Utility, Probability and Human Decision-making*. Reidel: Dordrecht.

Rasmussen, J. (1983). Skills, rules, and knowledge: Signals, signs, and symbols, and other distinctions in human performance models. *IEEE Transactions on Systems, Man, and Cybernetics*, SMC-13, 257–66.

Rasmussen, J. (1986). *Information Processing and Human–Machine Interaction: An Approach to Cognitive Engineering*. New York: North-Holland.

Rasmussen, J., Brehmer, B. and Leplat, L. (eds), (1991). *Distributed Decision-making: Cognitive Models for Cooperative Work*. Chichester: Wiley.

Rasmussen, J., Pejtersen, A.M. and Goodstein, L. (1994). *Cognitive Systems Engineering*. New York: Wiley.

Reason, J. (1997). *Managing the Risks of Organizational Accidents*. Aldershot: Ashgate.

Rencrantz, C., Lindoff, J., Svensson, E., Norlander, A. and Berggren, P. (2006). *Interoperability and Methodology Study in an Operative Command and Control Setting*. FOI–R–2040–SE, ISSN 1650–1942 (in Swedish).

Rochlin, G.I. (1997). *Trapped in the Net: The Unanticipated Consequences of Computerization*. Princeton, NJ: Princeton University Press.

Salas, E., Dickinson, T.L., Converse, S.A. and Tannenbaum, S.I. (1992). Towards an understanding of team performance and training. In R.W. Swezey and E. Salas (eds), *Teams: Their Training and Performance*. Norwood, NJ: Ablex Publishing Corporation, 3–30.

Senge, P.M. (1990). *The Fifth Discipline – The Art and Practice of the Learning Organization*. New York: Doubleday.

Serfaty, D. and Entin, E. (1997). Team adaptation and co-ordination training. In R. Flin, E. Salas, M. Strub and L. Martin (eds), *Decision-making Under Stress: Emerging Themes and Applications*. Aldershot: Ashgate.

Sheridan, T.B. (1997). Supervisory control. In G. Salvendy (ed.), *Handbook of Human Factors and Ergonomics*. New York: John Wiley & Sons.

Sjöberg, L., Svensson, E. and Persson, L.O. (1979). The measurement of mood. *Scandinavian Journal of Psychology*, 20, 1–18.

Smith, P., Woods, D.D., McCoy, E., Billings, C., Sarter, N., Denning, R. and Dekker S.W. (1997). *Human-centred Technologies and Procedures for Future Air Traffic Management*. Activities Report, Contract No. NAG2–995.

Svensson, E., Angelborg-Thandertz, M. and Sjöberg, L. (1993). Mission challenge, mental workload and performance in military aviation. *Aviation, Space and Environmental Medicine*, November, 985–91.

Svensson, E., Rencrantz, C., Lindoff, J., Berggren, P. and Norlander, A. (2006). Dynamic measures for performance assessment in complex environments. In *Proceedings of the Human Factors and Ergonomics Society 50th Annual Meeting*. Santa Monica, CA: The Human Factors Society.

Woods, D.D. and Roth, E.M. (1988). Cognitive engineering: Human problem solving with tools. *Human Factors*, 30, 415–30.

Worm, A. (1998a). Tactical joint cognitive systems performance in dynamic, distributed, time-critical operations. In *Proceedings of the 4th International Symposium on Command and Control Research and Technology*. Stockholm, Sweden.

Worm, A. (1998b). Joint tactical cognitive systems: Modelling, analysis, and performance assessment. In *Proceedings of the Human Factors and Ergonomics Society 42nd Annual Meeting*. Santa Monica, CA: The Human Factors Society.

Worm, A. (1998c). *Command and Control Science: Theory and Tactical Applications*. Linköping Studies in Science and Technology, Thesis No. 714, Linkoping University, Linkoping, Sweden.

Worm, A. (1999a). Mission efficiency analysis of tactical joint cognitive systems. In *Proceedings of the NATO International Symposium on Modelling and Analysis of Command and Control*. Paris, France.

Worm, A. (1999b). Evaluating tactical real-time interaction in multi-agent, dynamic, hazardous, high-stake operations. *In Proceedings of the Human Factors and Ergonomics Society 43rd Annual Meeting*. Santa Monica, CA: The Human Factors Society.

Worm, A. (2000a). *On Control and Interaction in Complex Distributed Systems and Environments*. Linköping Studies in Science and Technology, Dissertation No. 664, Linköping University, Linkoping, Sweden. ISBN 91–7219–899–0.

Worm, A. (2000b). Strategies for decision-making in complex systems control and mission command. In *Proceedings of the 5th Conference on Naturalistic Decision-making*. Stockholm, Sweden.

Worm, A. (2002). An integrated framework for information-centered human–machine systems analysis. *Int. J. Emergency Management*, 1(2), 125–43.

Worm, A., Jenvald, J. and Morin, M. (1998). Mission efficiency analysis: Evaluating and improving tactical mission performance in high-risk, time-critical operations. *Safety Science*, 30, 79–98. Elsevier Science B.V.

Zachary, W.W. and Ryder, J.M. (1997). Decision support systems: Integrating decision aiding and decision training. In M. Helander, T.K. Landauer and P. Prabhu (eds), *Handbook of Human–Computer Interaction*, 2nd edition. Amsterdam: Elsevier Science B.V.

Zeier, H. (1994). Workload and psychophysiological stress reactions in air traffic controllers. *Ergonomics*, 37, 525–39.

Zsambok, C.E. and Klein, G.A. (eds). (1997). *Naturalistic Decision-making*. Mahwah, NJ: Earlbaum.

Chapter 3

Designing Case Studies Using a Systems Analysis Approach

P. Wikberg

Introduction

This chapter outlines an approach to designing case studies based on systems analysis. The main argument is that a system analysis approach makes it possible to more efficiently make advances in a development process. The point of view is that the purpose of the system analysis is to explicitly translate relevant knowledge, assumptions, restrictions and expressed needs related to the problem in focus into problem statements and hypotheses expressed in terms of systems. The core of the system analysis approach is to produce a base for data collection about the stated problem, i.e. it should include a definition concerning how the measure should be conducted. The result of this problem analysis, or system analysis, represents the definition of the research design.

Given the increasing complexity and challenge of security environments worldwide, enormous pressure is being placed on ensuring warfighter performance readiness. Over the past decades, shrinking budgets and aging and/or inadequate Cold War defence systems have resulted in the need to increase efficient application of limited resources, yet maintain effectiveness (Paris et al. 2011). Consequently, and from a sheer pragmatic point, there is a need to test such solutions before implementation in order to have confidence in the procurement or implementation process. If test results are confounded, there is a risk of failed operations, loss of lives and money spent on inadequate solutions.

However, the possibility of testing every aspect of a solution in laboratories or on test benches is limited. When putting it all together, the 'system of system' effects of combining technology, people, procedures, organization, and so forth cannot be studied in a laboratory setting. The complexity is simply too great, and if too much control is imposed the dynamics of real operations are lost. It is often desirable or necessary to assess experts in their natural, dynamic environment, for example during a training session or a field exercise. It is rare to be allowed to interfere with active manipulations, and experimental control is not fully possible as the complexity is manifested in variables which exceed the number of available data points. In addition, it is seldom possible or suitable to have random assignment of participants to treatments, as organizational units must often be constructed according to considerations of training and experience. Consequently, it is difficult to fully apply the experimental method as conceived in science.

This is acknowledged by the military, and military experimentation is normally conducted in a much more complex setting compared to the settings used in traditional laboratory experiments. Tests are instead largely undertaken as what we, in this context, label 'case studies' (the term will be elaborated in the next section).

First, the concept of case studies will be elaborated. Then, some practical considerations and restrictions for conducting case studies are outlined as they are conceived in this context. This is followed by some basic considerations about systems analysis or modelling. Then, the approach of using systems analysis to design case studies is presented together with an illustrative case. The chapter is concluded with a discussion.

Case Studies

A case study is defined as 'an empirical inquiry that investigates a contemporary phenomenon within its real-life context when the boundaries between phenomenon and context are not clearly evident' (Yin 2003: 13). Being concerned with context in research practice is to introduce variables which exceed the number of available data points (Yin 2003). Still, multi-factor case studies assume that the system studied, irrespective of its complexity, has a reasonably simple structure which it is possible to study and evaluate. Compared to laboratory-based research, the case research method is based on the logic of analytical generalization and the experimentation isolation paradigm rather than on statistical generalization and the randomized-assignment-to-treatments model (Yin 2003; Silverman 2005). Theoretical replication is concerned with the construction of cases which are meaningful because they embrace criteria which are used to develop and test theoretically motivated, rival hypotheses (see also Mason 1996). The theoretically defined contrasts are translated into corresponding empirical contrasts. In general, the operationalization includes a set of multiple contingent factors, corresponding to a hypothetical pattern of criteria.

Consequently, the aim is not, as in natural science, to reveal general laws of nature. Instead it is about testing whether a specific solution is 'good enough' given existing possibilities and restrictions in technology, economy law, policies, and so forth. Conclusions are thus primarily for the given context, and the ambition is thus not necessarily for all circumstances. Similar to testing human–computer interaction solutions, the testing of organizational solutions implies a goal-oriented design process.

Another important consideration is that the way case studies are carried out has often been criticized. To quote Bromley (1986: xiii), 'case studies are sometimes carried out in a sloppy, perfunctory and incompetent manner and sometimes even in a corrupt, dishonest way'.

The position taken here is that the core concern is whether or not it is possible to implement appropriate checks to demonstrate reliability and validity in findings (Bromley 1986). The perspective here corresponds to Cook and Campbell's (1979: 79) notion that 'case studies should not be demeaned by identification with the one-group post-test-only design'. The full array of different designs should be considered in each and every case. Consequently, the content of this chapter refers to rigorous case study designs involving matters of problem analysis, data collection, analysis, interpretation and communication of results.

The practical implication of having studies with more variables than available data points is that the conclusions cannot be based on deductive logic. Even with the most carefully prepared design, there will always be factors present which might have biased the result. This is exactly the reason why theoretical considerations are of such importance when designing multi-factor case studies. A carefully defined model supported by an array of triangulated indices forms the basis for an analytical generalization. The line of proof resembles that of a court trial in which there is no technical evidence. The prosecutor has to base his case on a set of indices which, taken together, form a comprehensive pattern making it plausible enough for a verdict of guilty. Similarly, the analyst must be able to present a case in which theoretical considerations are supported by empirical indices in a comprehensive way, thus making it 'good enough' as a basis for decisions on the systems of systems in focus.

This approach uses systems analysis to define such models.

Systems Analysis

There are several definitions of the term 'systems analysis', but any definition usually involves some kind of procedure, more or less formal, for collecting and organizing data about an empirical phenomenon into a system model. There are a variety of systems analysis techniques and approaches, such as 'task analysis' (Annett et al. 1971; Drury et al. 1987), 'job analysis' (Harvey 1991), 'content analysis' (Weber 1990; Kolbe 1991), 'action analysis' (Singleton 1979) and 'cognitive systems engineering' (Hollnagel and Woods 1983; Rasmussen et al. 1994). Despite the fact that these techniques differ somewhat when it comes to perspectives and procedures, they are rather similar. They are related to a scientific style of approaching a certain phenomenon analytically, in order to treat or analyse reality as a systematically connected set of elements (Gasparski 1991).

By definition, a model is a real or imaginary representation of a real system. The basic logic of a model is analogy in terms of patterns of similarity and differences between the model and the subject for the system analysis (Harré 2002). By reducing the complexity of reality but still containing relevant information, the model might be used as a tool, a schema or a procedure to predict the consequences of an event. The properties of a model will be formally defined as a set of elements or conceptual terms, a set of rules for relations between the elements, a set of empirical elements and relations corresponding to the conceptual terms and relations and, finally, a set of rules for interpretation.

The Systems Analysis Procedure

In a more general sense, the system analysis process might be a serial and additive effort of instantiating specific plans or using analogical transformations to known solutions of similar problems, if the problem to be modelled is well structured (Carbonell 1986). However, as the problem to be solved in system analysis is often ill structured, the process is presumably better characterized as an iterative, non-linear interaction between overlapping and fuzzy domains. In addition, the problem domain which is to be modelled is often too complex for a single expert to master. Thus, it is often necessary to engage different individuals in a team effort in the system analysis enterprise. Each of the participants is supposed to bring their specific competence and knowledge to the model. At a minimum, the system analysis enterprise engages two persons, the analyst and the respondent. The model is constructed in an interactive process between these individuals. Consequently, the system analysis procedure might be viewed as a group process. Coordinating the process – problem solving over time – is an important aspect for group performance (Paulus 2000). The level of control of the interactive process varies between different system analysis techniques. A rough classification of system analysis procedures can be based on the extremes in terms of level of control: system analysis based on information from independent respondents and system analysis in teams (Wikberg 2007).

Independent participants or one-participant system analysis
In this case, the analyst is interacting with one participant at a time. The basic procedure is to first let different participants contribute independently to the system analysis, and then synthesize a solution. Consequently, the end product evolves successively as different models are contrasted against each other. The group factor is controlled by independent sampling and of course by a standardized procedure. The analyst will have a great impact on the end result, as he will largely define the procedure of bringing different model representations into line with each other.

Interdependent participants or team system analysis
In this case the system analysis team consists of several participants interacting in a group effort. The basic procedure is to let the model successively evolve in the interaction between different participants. Synthesizing an end result is then embedded in the data elicitation procedure. The group factor is a part of the design of the system analysis procedure. The process is, however, not solely about objectively piecing together knowledge. The process is highly social and all the participants' objective levels of expertise, as well as the extent to which their expertise is recognized, will have an effect on this interaction (Littlepage and Mueller 1997; Bromme et al. 2001).

At this point it should again be noted that the initial system analysis is not equivalent to empirical testing. Instead, the purpose is normally to create a foundation for a practical application such as a system solution or a complex case study design. In order to achieve this outcome the system analysis must have some specific characteristics.

The Expected Outcome of the System Analysis Procedure

The general expected outcome of the system analysis procedure is one or several system models.

System thinking views the world as a complex system of interconnected entities where 'everything affects everything'. The system components are interrelated and interdependent and cannot exist independently. However, neither in practice nor in theory is it possible to take all these entities into consideration when a problem or phenomenon is analysed or described. Instead, the most relevant interactions and entities are defined as being inside the system boundary. Entities outside the system boundary are still recognized as having the potential to influence the system but are viewed as a part of the system's environment. The environment is described as simplified representations or models of the actual system.

One way of describing this reduction is to use a bull's-eye diagram where the entities or interactions of a system are divided into three categories depending on how important they are for describing the system and how relevant they are for answering the question(s) the system model tries to illuminate. The entities that are inside the system boundary are called endogenous; in the model they can influence other entities as well as be influenced by other endogenous entities. The entities that belong to the environment of the system are called exogenous; they can influence endogenous entities but are not influenced by other entities themselves. The least relevant entities are excluded from the model altogether and do not therefore have any influence on the entities in the system model. These three categories are shown in Figure 3.1.

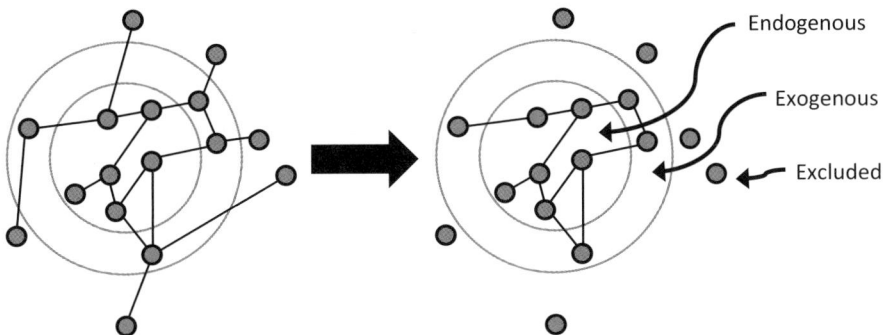

Figure 3.1   Bull's-eye diagram

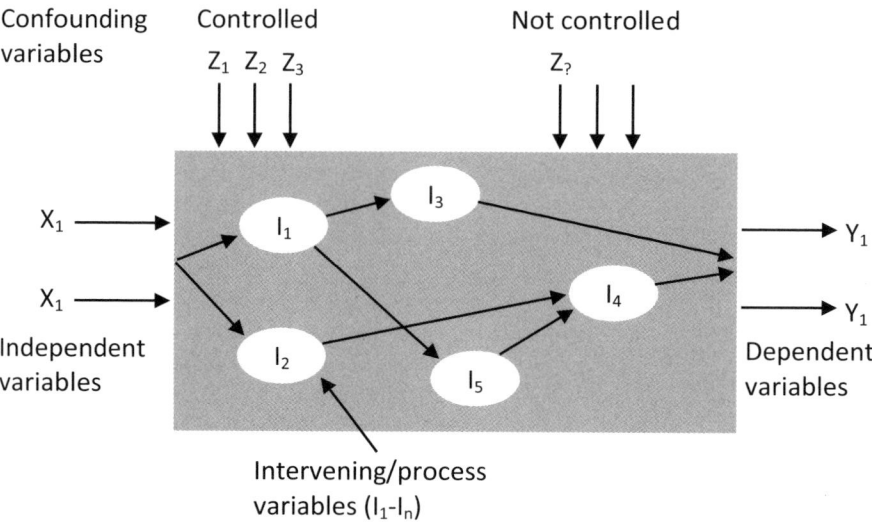

Figure 3.2   A general systems model
Source: From Strangert (2006). Adapted by permission of the author.

In the context of experiments, general systems theory defines subsets of different variables: input variables causing an effect on the system (independent variables), output variables representing the overall effect on the system (dependent variables), and process variables representing factors that explain the relationship between cause and effect (intervening or process variables). These variables are shown in Figure 3.2.

Case studies, as experiments or similar tests, require a procedure for assessment. In order to assess a model, such as the one in Figure 3.2, some conditions have to be met (Wikberg 1997): (a) there must be a set of elements, conceptual terms, explicitly defined; (b) there must be a set of defined formal rules for relations between the elements which determine the possible combinations; and (c) there must be a set of defined empirical elements and relations corresponding to the model.

It is possible to map empirical relational structures into formal qualitative relational structures. For example, any ethnic language can be seen as a natural representation system to represent thoughts, happenings, processes, etc. The language as a representation system has different objects (words) and rules for relations (grammar) which are intended to represent and describe reality. The ethnic language can be translated to other ethnic languages as well as to formal predicate logic. If the empirical relation has a high degree of uniqueness, the number of possible transformations decreases. Based on this assumption, the distinction between quantitative and qualitative research is somewhat blurred as any given reality can be represented by a large or even infinitive number of models (Silverman 2001).

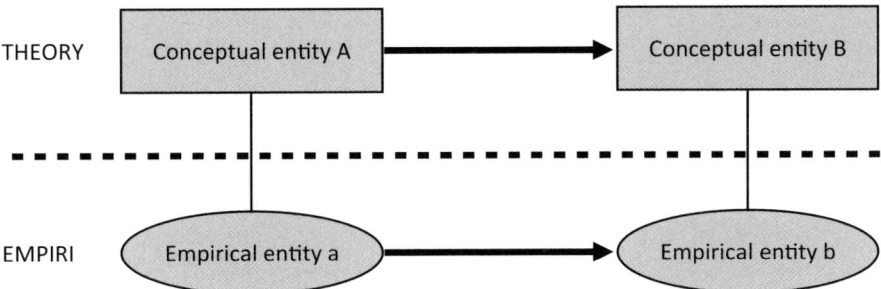

Figure 3.3   A conceptual cause and effect model with corresponding empirical entities

The model in Figure 3.2 can be developed to illustrate the connection between the model's conceptual elements and the corresponding empirical entities, as shown in Figure 3.3.

Formal measurement theory (Krantz et al. 1971) suggests two theorems: the representation theorem and the uniqueness theorem.

The representation theorem
If a specific structure of relations in an empirical system is measurable it is possible to make a homomorphic reproduction of that empirical system into a formal and numerical system. Several different specific empirical objects can be represented according to the theorem by one single numerical value or class. Several different objects can be related to a summarizing category in order to express a certain quality that the different terms are judged to have in common. For example, a large number of individuals may be categorized into a fewer number of categories, such as 'expert' and 'non-expert'.

Another related notion in measurement theory is the distinction between four different scales of measurements (Stevens 1946). Scale type is important because it defines which types of relations can be preserved in a measurement operation, but not all relations can be represented using a certain measurement scale. It is possible to represent reality in a number of ways. For example, a military unit can be represented numerically according to several principles: level of protection, level of training, command structure, etc.

The uniqueness theorem
The representation theorem calls for the relational structure in a chosen representation system to correspond to the relational structure in the empirical system. This puts a limit on the possible transformations between different representational models. The uniqueness theorem states that every empirical relation has only a few appropriate ways of representing a numerical model.

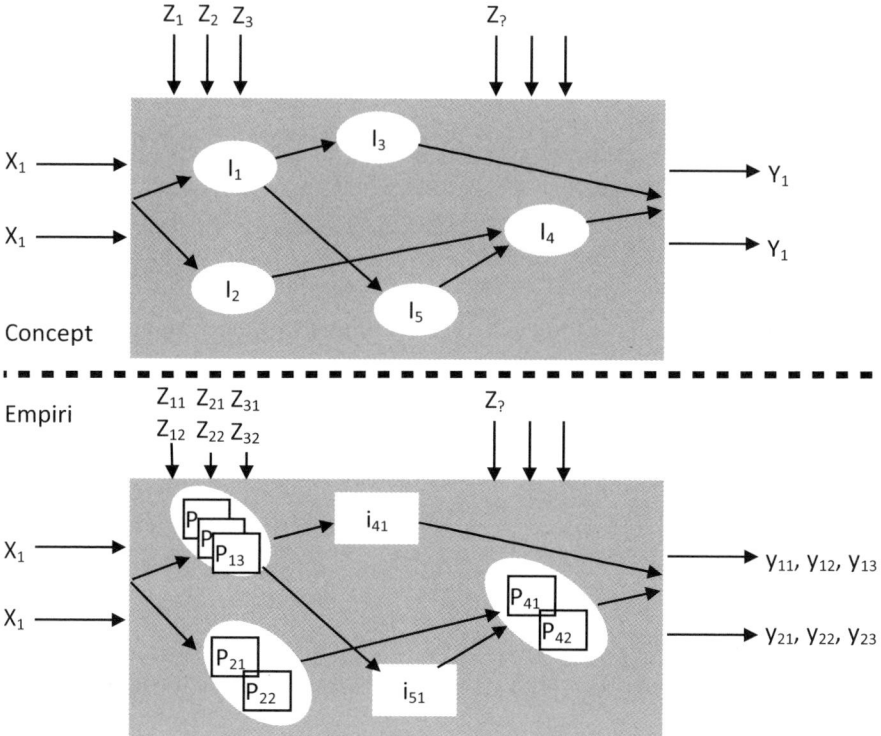

Figure 3.4   A model of correspondence between conceptual and empirical levels

Source: From Strangert (2006). Adapted by permission of the author.

Krantz et al. (1971) discuss numerical representation, but other types of representation are possible, for example those based on semantics or predicate logics (Flood and Carson 1990). Subjective judgements can be represented by a quantitative scale or by qualitative descriptions using natural language (Strangert 2006).

When designing case studies using a systems analysis approach it is vital that stakeholders participate in the process of designing the case study as well as selecting measures and representations. The evaluation model must be specified to enable empirical assessment, i.e., empirical elements and the relations between them that correspond to the model's conceptual terms must be specified. This is illustrated in Figure 3.4.

The conceptual elements $(X_1-X_n, I_1-I_n, Z_1-Z_n, Y_1-Y_n)$ are representations of a set of corresponding empirical indices $(x_1-x_n,$ etc.) which it is possible to measure, or at least implement at the nominal scale level. Each conceptual element should represent several empirical elements (such as I1 representing the empirical elements p_{11}, p_{12} and p_{13}). Some conceptual elements cannot be measured directly and must thus be theoretically assumed and measured indirectly (such as I_4 measured indirectly by i_{41}).

In a design task the model representing the 'system of system' solution will have a limited validity over time and between settings. This has implications on the conceptual as well as the empirical level. The conceptual model should include current scientific knowledge. It can also include factors such as policies, available technology, economic realities and other regulations and restrictions. The life cycles for these factors are limited. Further, system of systems solutions that are successfully implemented in one environment might be completely inappropriate in another. Not only will the success of the implemented solution vary between environments, but also the meaning of the data obtained from the measurements will vary.

Information Sources for Systems Analysis

The full array of information sources should be considered. The characteristics of the task will define or constrain appropriate methods for eliciting information (Hoffman et al. 1995). Based on a preliminary task analysis, the system analysis task should be structured theoretically and a procedure for the systems analysis should be defined. Relevant knowledge domains, basic model structure, important restrictions, and so on, form the basis for definitions of which information sources to include.

Roles in the Systems Analysis Procedure

It is possible to identify different roles for the individuals participating in a systems analysis enterprise (Wikberg 2007). An analyst, whose task is to coordinate the session, may manage the system analysis. A domain expert is an individual who has developed knowledge and abilities in a certain area. A domain is an abstract or physical phenomenon in which it is possible to define specific knowledge and abilities. The system user or end user has a special case of domain expertise, i.e. specific knowledge of how the system analysis subject would be used in a real context.

Design of Case Studies through Systems Analysis

System analysis of case study design often needs two major types of model. The first type is a business model which describes the organization, technology or process which is the framework for the case study. The second type is a measurement model which defines the relevant factors to be measured, i.e. an operational definition of the actual research question. However, the distinction between the models is not always clear. The model types are rather to be seen as complementary perspectives.

Business Models

The business model is intended to give an outline of participants and systems included in the experiment, the relation between them and the systems' input and output. The main purpose is to specify the context in which the experiment is conducted.

The test environment should as much as possible be represented by real systems and real personnel. An experimental situation might, of course, include other essential aspects not described in the model, for example a tactical situation or a staff supporting the commander. What to include in the business model, and thereby in the experimentation or simulation, is dependent on the situation and setting.

Measurement Models

A business model is not enough as a foundation for experimental design; there are also expectations about the outcome. These expectations, in the form of hypotheses, should be included in a measurement model. The purpose of this model is to define hypotheses and/or research questions. As in the case of the business model it is essential that the manifestation, or operationalization, of the elements in the model is defined. The elements in the model constitute the construction of instruments for measurement. The measurement model is basically a hypothesis tree with a number of generic elements – see Figure 3.5.

Independent variable (X)
It is possible to compare different organizational or technological solutions. An independent variable could be new work method compared to old work method.

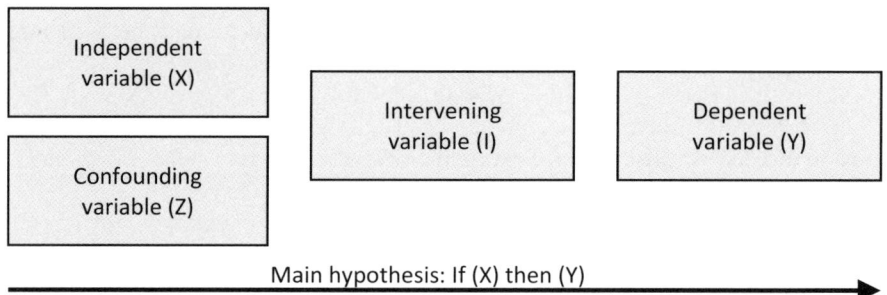

Figure 3.5   A generic measurement model

Dependent variable (Y)
What differences in performance will the new organizational or technological solution impose? As a result of the variation between conditions the dependent variables are expected to vary.

Confounding variable (Z)
It is not possible to create exactly equivalent conditions for all aspects in case studies. Variables other than the independent variable that affect the dependent variable and consequently confound the result must be controlled for by elimination, minimization, held constant or explicitly randomized.

Intervening variable (I)
There might exist other processes or variables that are affected by the independent variable, which in turn affect the dependent variable. The intervening variable might affect the dependent variable differently for different circumstances surrounding the independent variable. Therefore, it is important to identify and understand the intervening variable.

Hypotheses
The model also presents the hypothesis to be tested. The main hypothesis is the (proposed) relationship between the independent and dependent variables. It is also possible to define explanatory hypotheses which describe the influence of the intervening variable.

An Example of Designing a Case Study

In this section an example of a systems analysis approach to designing a case study is presented (Wikberg et al. 2004). In this study two different training environments for the command and control (C2) of Ranger units were compared. One setting was a real physical environment. The other setting was a virtual PC game environment. The research question was to compare these two settings. Is it possible to use a simulated environment in combination with real C2 systems to train Ranger units?

The units' and the commander's execution of the mission in the two different environments were compared according to mission success, communication, situation awareness and the dynamics of the task. Data were gathered using observers, questionnaires and recording of radio communication.

Business Model

With support from military personnel from the Army's Ranger Battalion (K4), a business model of command and control for Ranger units was defined – see Figure 3.6 for the case of reconnaissance data from an unmanned aerial vehicle (UAV). The realization of the model in the two different settings is presented in Table 3.1.

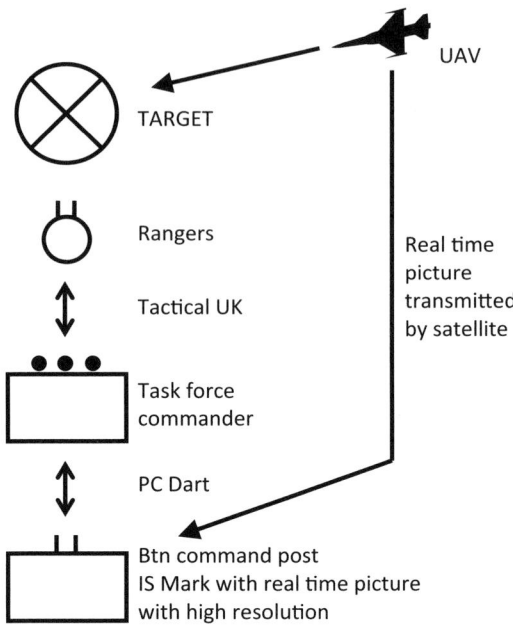

Figure 3.6   A business model of the command and control organization when real-time information from a UAV is available

Table 3.1   Description of the elements in the business model and how these were realized in each setting

Model Elements	Description
Target	Objects, activities or area which constitutes the task force's mission. *Realized by:* The objective was to demolish a communication pylon. In the physical setting the pylon was located about 50 metres south of a building present in the mission area. The pylon was replicated in the virtual setting.
Rangers	The Ranger unit; part of the task force with the task of striking at the objective. *Realized by:* Conscripts from the 41st Ranger platoon. In the physical setting weapons rigged for blank ammunition and blind explosives were used. The soldiers were equipped with equipment to indicate gunfire using laser indicators. In the virtual setting each soldier had access to a computer connected to the LAN and each of them controlled one player.
Task force commander	The individual commanding the mission in the field. In missions concerning few units the task commander normally is in close connection to the soldiers at the objective. In missions with several units the location most suitable for the coordination of the mission is chosen. *Realized by:* Consisted of conscripts from 41st Ranger platoon. These were using the same equipment as the other soldiers in both settings.

Model Elements	Description
Tactical radio communication	Within the task force the communication between units is based on a radio UHF system. *Realized by:* The ordinary radio system was used in both settings.
Btn command post	The battalion command located at a rear command post has the task of supporting the task commander. *Realized by:* Officers from the regiment with the rank of captain. That position was in accordance with the position they would have during a real operation. The rear command post in the virtual setting consisted of one officer located in the facility used as the rear command post during the regiment's regular exercises. The rear command post in the physical setting was located in a hut not far from the physical mission area. Both rear command posts had the same access to command and control support systems.
PC DART	A long-range communication system based on HF radio and a PC-based terminal for communicating data. *Realized by:* In communications between the mission and the rear command post the Radio 180 was used in both the real and virtual settings.
UAV/real-time image via satellite	A sensor. In this particular case defined as a UAV able to register activities in the mission area in real time. *Realized by:* The real-time information from the UAV in the virtual setting was an existing functionality of the PC game used. The UAV picture was presented on a screen on a terminal connected to the local network in the rear command post. The UAV could be controlled by the task force commander. The picture was not available to the task force. In the physical setting a remote-controlled web camera was mounted on a skylift placed in the mission area. In accordance with the virtual setting the commander in the physical setting could control the view of the simulated UAV. Furthermore, the picture from the web camera was not available to the task force. The position and altitude of the simulated UAV function was as equal as possible in both settings.

Measurement Model

There were two major expectations regarding the outcome. (1) There might be a difference between settings regarding mission performance. (2) There might also be an order effect, that is, an effect on mission performance due to which setting is first executed.

Mission performance was assumed to be reflected in both the performance of the task force and the performance of the command post. Task force performance was reflected in whether the task was solved or not (demolish the communication pylon without losses), time to accomplish mission, expressed preparedness to adapt to alternatives, level of risk taking and tactically correct behaviour as judged by training officers. Similarly, command post performance was reflected in the ability to deliver correct and adequate information as judged by task forces and training officers, and correspondence in perception of task force activity between command

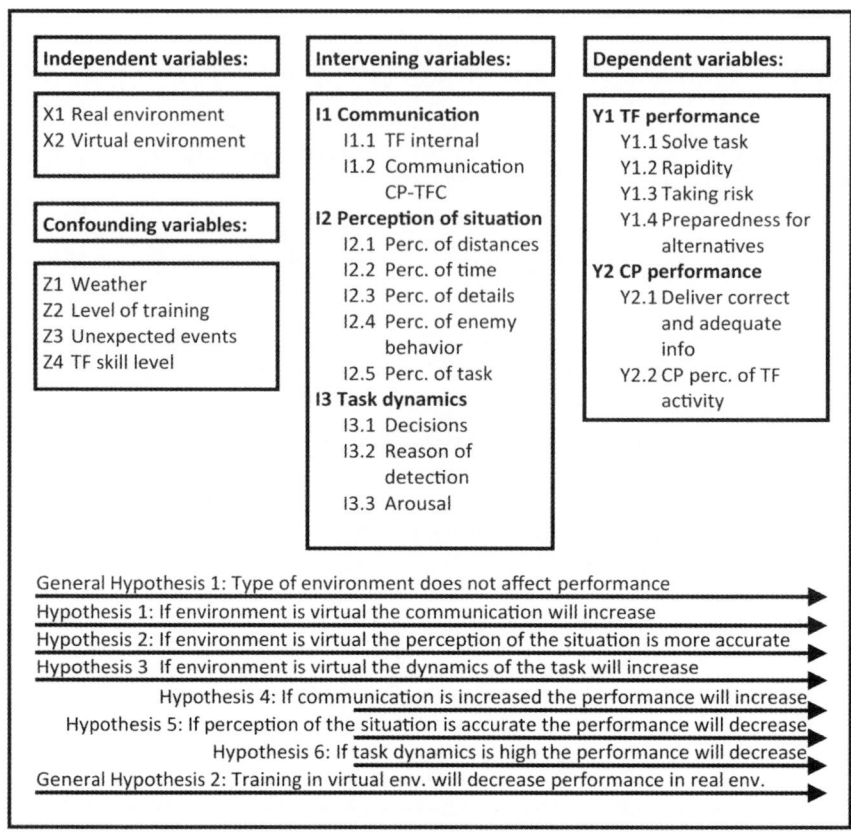

Figure 3.7   Measurement model for the Ranger case study

post and training officer. These expectations were transformed into a measurement model with a set of interconnected hypotheses, as shown in Figure 3.7.

The measurement model corresponds to the major expectations outlined earlier in this section. It defines two major dependent variables, task force performance and command post performance, that might be affected between the two settings. Each of these variables consists of a set of sub-variables. Some intervening variables where identified as possible explanations to variation in the dependent variable. Finally, some confounding variables were also identified, including weather and task force skill level. Therefore, these factors were also monitored.

The results from the study revealed that the task forces' performance and behaviour were more or less the same in the different settings. However, it should be noted that communication within task forces was more frequent and different in character in the virtual environment. Furthermore, the communication between commander and task force was more frequent in the real environment.

The outcome of the exercise lent support to the continuation of the study with a more advanced and complex experiment.

Discussion

This chapter aimed at presenting an approach to designing case studies based on a systems analysis perspective. The main argument is that the approach overcomes some of the problems 'normal science' has in supporting development processes. The heuristic modelling approach makes it possible to make advances more efficiently in a development process.

No formalized procedure has been presented. This is intentional. The position taken here is that the procedure should be defined specifically for each case. It is also important to note that the number and complexity of the models needed for a case study design might vary. Procedures might be developed for specific problem areas, but in that case such procedures are often already in place. The perspective here is multidisciplinary. Depending on the knowledge domains involved, the available resources, time frames, etc. the specific procedures might vary. Instead, the procedure should be anchored in the characteristics of the expected outcome. Correspondingly, the case used to illustrate the approach was selected due to its relative simplicity. It should only be viewed as an example.

Applying a case study approach in complex development endeavours calls for a slightly different perspective compared to normal science. In this context, the aim is not always generalized knowledge valid in all relevant situations. Constructed systems such as organizations or procedures are subject to constant change. Introduction of new equipment or even replacement of individuals might substantially change preconditions and system behaviour, and thus the validity of earlier assessments of the system. In many cases, therefore, the validity of a case study is limited in time and target population. Thus, the important consideration is to assess the validity of the case study in the context of the aim of the development process (often initiated by a real need to solve a practical problem).

The remarks above raise the question of whether case studies in the context of practical development processes qualify to be labelled as 'science' – part of the demarcation problem (Shermer 2001) which is about how and where to draw the lines around science. Science is one of mankind's most important tools for development. As a general rule it should be considered important to keep the term science clean from con artists.

Still, science has problems dealing with issues concerning systems of systems. Although mainstream science in some areas has been extremely successful, other areas show little or no real progress, especially when humans and human behaviour are important features of the system studied. The response on these problems in terms of alternative approaches (hermeneutics and related approaches) has arguably not performed any better. Scientific knowledge in terms of explanation and prediction of system behaviour is normally poor or at too high a level to translate to the specific situation or problem. As a contrast, in the somewhat parallel universe of the art of engineering, it is easier to find success stories. Although working with solutions based on principles uncovered by science, engineering also implements other aspects, some of them even controversial from an assessment perspective such as aesthetical properties, into workable solutions.

The position here is that the question cannot be answered in a general sense. Instead, each separate case study should be judged individually. Some will, perhaps due to favourable conditions, qualify for the criteria of science, i.e. in practice can be published in a peer-reviewed format. Others will not. The core point is that validity of findings is as important in the complex development project as in the scientific project. The consequences of failed practical development projects might often be substantially more severe. In contrast, failure to find support for a hypothesis in a scientific project is as important for knowledge development as success in finding support. Consequently, carefully designed studies are as important in a practical project as in science.

Note that the dichotomy between scientific projects and practical projects indicated above is arbitrary and far from distinct. In practice they should perhaps not be contrasted with each other. A practical project might include an array of activities based on dogmatic scientific practice. Each of them might contribute, alone or taken together, with valuable inputs for the end result in terms of the practical aim of the project. Similarly, experiences from a practical project might provide valuable inputs to general scientific knowledge.

One potential distinction between the practical project and the scientific project is that the practical project must normally accept more uncertainty in their decisions on how to proceed (or rather in the final decision on how to design the end product). System tests or assessments, i.e. case studies, are an important basis for taking these decisions. Knowledge of the limitations of system assessments is thus important. Consequently, personnel acquainted with the principles and practices of science are a valuable resource in a complex development project. The systems analysis approach to designing the case studies is a potential tool to coordinate development activities in such a fashion that the validity of findings can be assessed both from a practical perspective and from a scientific perspective to reveal strengths and shortcomings.

References

Annett, J., Duncan, D., Stammers, R.B. and Gray, M.J. (1971). *Task Analysis*. London: Her Majesty's Stationary Office.

Bromley, D.B. (1986). *The Case Study Method in Psychology and Related Disciplines*. Chichester: Wiley.

Bromme, R., Rambow, R. and Nückles, M. (2001). Expertise and estimating what other people know: The influence of professional experience and type of knowledge. *Journal of Experimental Psychology: Applied*, 7(4), 317–30.

Carbonell, J.G. (1986). Derivational analogy: A theory of reconstructive problem solving and expertise acquisition. In R.S. Michalski, J.G. Carbonell and T.M. Mitchell (eds), *Machine Learning II: An Artificial Intelligence Approach*. Los Altos, CA: Morgan Kauffman, 371–92.

Cook, T.D. and Campbell, D.T. (1979). *Quasi-Experimentation: Design and Analysis for Field Settings*. Chicago, IL: Rand McNally.

Drury, C.G., Paramore, B., Van Cott, H.P., Grey, S.M. and Corlett, E.N. (1987). Task analysis. In G. Salvendy (ed.), *Handbook of Human Factors*. New York: John Wiley & Sons, 370–401.

Flood, R.L. and Carson, E.R. (1990). *Dealing with Complexity*. New York: Plenum Press.

Gasparski, W.W. (1991). Systems approach as a style: A hermeneutics of systems. In M.C. Jackson, G.J. Mansell, R.L. Flood, R.B. Blackham and S.V.E. Probert (eds), *Systems Thinking in Europe*. New York: Plenum Press, 15–27.

Harré, R. (2002). *Cognitive Science: A Philosophical Introduction*. London: Sage.

Harvey, R.J. (1991). Job analysis. In M.D. Dunnette and L.M. Hough (eds), *Handbook of Industrial and Organisational Psychology*, 2nd ed., vol. 2. Palo Alto, CA: Consulting Psychologists Press, Inc., 71–163.

Hoffman, R.R., Shadbolt, N.R., Burton, A.M. and Klein, G. (1995). Eliciting knowledge from experts: A methodological analysis. *Organizational Behavior and Human Decision Processes*, 62(2), 129–58.

Hollnagel, E. and Woods, D.D. (1983). Cognitive systems engineering: New wine in new bottles. *International Journal of Man-Machine Studies*, 18, 583–600.

Kolbe, R.H. (1991). Content analysis research: An examination of applications with directives for improving research reliability and objectivity. *Journal of Consumer Research*, 18, 243–50.

Krantz, D., Luce, R.D., Suppes, P. and Tversky, A. (1971). *Foundations of Measurement*, vol. 1. San Diego: Academic Press, 1–33.

Littlepage, G.E. and Mueller, A.L. (1997). Recognition and utilization of expertise in problem solving groups: Expert characteristics and behavior. *Group Dynamics: Theory, Research and Practice*, 1(4), 324–8.

Mason, J. (1996). *Qualitative Researching*. London: Sage.

Paris, C., Banko, K., Berggren, P., Burov, A., Davis, K., Halpin, S., Kermarrec, Y., Lussier, J., Quiram, T., Schaab, B., Ward, J. and Wikberg, P. (2011). *Measuring and Analyzing Command and Control Performance Effectiveness*. NATO RTO Technical Report TR-HFM-156.

Paulus, P.B. (2000). Groups, teams, and creativity: The creative potential of idea-generating groups. *Applied Psychology: An International Review*, 49(2), 237–62.

Rasmussen, J., Pejtersen, A.M. and Goodstein, L.P. (1994). *Cognitive Systems Engineering*. New York: Wiley.

Shermer, M. (2001). *The Borderlands of Science: Where Sense Meets Nonsense*. New York: Oxford University Press.

Silverman, D. (2001). *Interpreting Qualitative Data. Methods for Analyzing Talk, Text and Interaction*, 2nd ed. London: Sage.

Silverman, D. (2005). *Doing Qualitative Research*, 2nd ed. London: Sage.

Singleton, W.T. (ed.). (1979). *The Study of Real Skills. Compliance and Excellence*, vol. 2. Lancaster: MTP.

Stevens, S.S. (1946). On the theory of scales and measurement. *Science*, 103, 677–80.

Strangert, B. (2006). *Försöksmetodik för utvecklingsansvariga i Försvarsmakten*. Available at http://www.arborg.se/arkiv/forsoksmetodik2006 [accessed 9 February 2014].

Weber, R.P. (1990). *Basic Content Analysis*, 2nd ed. Beverly Hills, CA: Sage.

Wikberg, P. (1997). *Using Expert Descriptions in Systems Analysis*. Licentiate Thesis, University of Umeå: Department of Psychology.

Wikberg, P. (2007). *Eliciting Knowledge from Experts in Modeling of Complex Systems: Managing Variation and Interactions*. Department of Computer and Information Science, Linköping Studies in Science and Technology, Doctoral Dissertation Thesis No 1139. Linköping, Sweden: Linköping University.

Wikberg, P., Andersson, J., Berggren, J., Hedström, J., Lindoff, J., Rencrantz, C., Thorstensson, M. and Holmström, H. (2004). *Simulerade Insatsmiljöer i Kommersiella PC-spel som Försöksplattformar. Skillnader mellan Genomförande av Jägarinsats i en Virtuell Miljö med ett Genomförande i Riktig Terräng med Lös Ammunition och Simfireutrustning*. Metodrapport, FOI-R--1416—SE.

Yin, R.K. (2003). *Case Study Research. Design and Methods*, 3rd ed. London: Sage.

Chapter 4
Dynamic Measures of Effectiveness in Command and Control

E. Svensson and S. Nählinder

Introduction

In the following, we promote state of the art measures that capture dynamic changes and variances over time in typical command and control environments. The so-called old way is contrasted with the new way of interpreting data, hence differences regarding questions that can be answered. Variance and change are basic aspects of experimentation and measurement. The importance of inter- and intra-individual sources of variance, as well as their impact on covariation between variables, will be explained and emphasized. The components of repeated measures or time series (levels or mean value, long-term movements and seasonal vs periodical changes) are explained. Statistical considerations, such as stationarity with respect to systematic trends, variance constancy of variables and constancy of covariance over time of time series or repeated measures, are discussed and examples presented. Techniques for transformation and smoothing of time series, modelling and forecasting are demonstrated; *dynamic factor analysis* (DFA) is a statistical technique for analysis and reduction of a larger number of manifest time series variables to a smaller set of dynamic factors. The technique and modelling of DFA is illustrated by means of *structural equation modelling* (SEM). Practicable techniques for dynamic measurement are demonstrated, and the predictive power of DFA illustrated.

Measurement Theory and Statistical Techniques

Psychological measurement captures, reflects, a status or condition of an individual at a certain moment, or during a given (predetermined) time sequence (for example mental workload or situational awareness at a specific occasion or during a mission). Measures of this type of information can be argued to be static because they represent a momentary condition, or an average of a condition or state, over a time sequence. However, most operational situations like command and control environments are dynamic and complex settings with interacting systems and teams of operators. It is reasonable to assume that these settings represent interacting and interdependent processes; measures of momentary or average conditions over time are simply insufficient and/or inappropriate as representations of these processes. Further, it can be assumed that the variation of these processes over time is a function of both preceding and actual internal (psychological) and external (situational) conditions. As will be shown, such dependencies are crucial for modelling, as well as for the prediction of future conditions and states.

Most statistical techniques used in human factors research are based on inter-individual variation generated by independent measures from a large number of participants; inferences at population level are made from differences between participants at sample level. However, in the settings focused on here, every operator forms some part of the (series of) processes that push a process forward. It is exactly this variation among participants, over time and situation, which is of critical importance. It has been pointed out by Molenaar that 'inferred states of affairs at the population level do not apply at the level of intra-individual variation characterizing the life trajectories of individual participants making up the population' (Molenaar 2006; Molenaar and Ram 2010). Molenaar also emphasizes the importance of the intra-individual variation in terms of time series measures and the need for alternative statistical approaches such as dynamic factor analysis (DFA) in studies of situations such as the ones discussed here.

In human factors research, the systems approach has primarily been devoted to technical aspects, but in studies of man–system interaction (MSI), the systems approach may be attributed to human aspects as well (van Geert and van Dijk 2002; Boff 2006). Accordingly, an operator is seen as a multidimensional dynamic system with interacting subsystems, the behaviour of which changes as a function of internal and external influences over time. The use of dynamic systems methodology to describe intra-individual variability is considered to be a promising area of research (Bertenthal 2007; Deboeck and Boker 2010).

Time series can be defined as measures reflecting individual dynamic changes or processes over shorter or longer periods of time; a time series is a sequence of observations made over time. Differences between consecutive observations reflect intra-individual variability. Time series are common in a variety of fields from, for example, economics, physiology, psychology and engineering (Chatfield 2004). In behavioural research, time series of psychophysiological variables (for example heart and brain activity) and responses to questionnaire items (concerning, for instance, workload, situational awareness and performance) have been used in the modelling of human performance (Angelborg-Thanderz 1997; Svensson et al. 1997a; Berggren 2000, 2005; Svensson and Wilson 2002; Nählinder et al. 2004; Svensson et al. 2006; Nählinder 2009; Svensson et al. 2013).

Time series of psychophysiological variables are mostly continuous, while time series of, for example, responses to questionnaires are discrete. A time series is argued to be continuous when measures are taken continuously; it is discrete when measures are taken only at specific occasions. It is important to notice that a discrete time series can (and often does) represent a genuine continuous variable. Repeated questions at ordinal level of genuinely continuous psychological variables such as mental workload, situational awareness and performance are examples of discrete time series and often called quasi-dynamic (Svensson et al. 1997a, 2006). (The practical use of this type of time series is illustrated in Chapter 7 of this volume.)

Time series of psychophysiological measures (heart rate, for instance) have long been used for monitoring states such as, for example, operator mental workload (Caldwell et al. 1994; Svensson and Wilson 2002; Wilson et al. 2004). Psychological time series measures like repeated questionnaires have been used in studies of mood structures and changes (Shifren et al. 1997) and also in studies of affective processes (Ferrer and Nesselroade 2003).

Measuring psychophysiological variables tends to be unobtrusive, while asking for answers through questionnaires requires the participants' attention, something which may interfere with behaviour and cognitive performance. In this respect, questionnaire answers can be compared to secondary task techniques that are used in human factors research. Questionnaire answers may, further, be integrated as elements in operators' behavioural processes.

In most command and control studies, changes that occur over minutes, hours or days are of interest, so called transient fluctuations. Slower changes (over months and years) are looked upon as systematic trends (Nesselroade 1991). Learning and skill acquisition, to mention a couple of examples, are relatively slow processes and thereby represent systematic trends (Browne and Zhang 2007).

As noted above, measures can reflect a status at a certain time, or they can explore, mirror, more dynamic changes. The measurements complement each other and reflect different aspects of, for example, command and control processes, although capturing the dynamic changes of a command and control situation can be an endeavour more challenging than noting stable or slow change situations. Dynamic changes, however, provide information that cannot be gained through traditional measures merely focusing on static aspects of situations.

Repeated measurement techniques are of imperative importance for predicting changes concerning complex and dynamic events in command and control environments. Through predictions of changes in mental workload, early adaptive changes in performance by teams, sub-teams and positions can be carried out.

Variation and Change

Change, variation, is the foundation of experimental science. Without varying phenomena, relations cannot be identified, thus no conclusions about differences drawn. If two or more phenomena vary (that is, constitute variables) and they vary in systematic and concordant ways, there are covariances or inter-correlations between these variables. Classical statistics concerns experimentation with comparisons and tests of differences and changes; multivariate statistics concerns covariations and techniques such as *factor analysis* (FA) and *structural equation modelling* (SEM).

In spite of the fact that most psychological phenomena change over time and this change in itself is of importance, experiences from studies of dynamic systems has so far had little impact on the psychological sciences (Bertenthal 2007).

Inter-Individual Variability and Classical Experimentation Designs

Differences between cases or individuals constitute the main source of data variability in classical statistical analyses within the field of behavioural experimentation. The inter-individual variability of independent measures from a sample of participants forms a base for inferences at population level. Measurement errors that tend to occur are random and independent of true values, and symmetrically distributed around true values; they are also reduced as the number of participants increases.

Typically, numerous cases are measured after two or more different treatments. For example, participants' performance can be compared between different types of training, or when systems of different designs are used. In these cases, differences induced by different treatment conditions are compared and probabilities for statistically significant differences are calculated. However, probability values only indicate whether different treatments have had significant effects on performance – or not. They do not say anything about the size of the effect on performance. In analyses of data with high statistical power (studies with a large number of participants in each treatment group), significant differences are generated even if the differences in performance between the groups are small and thereby have limited practical importance. For this reason, classical experimental designs and statistics based on inter-individual variance have restricted explanatory power.

For situations like command and control environments, classical experimental design is less appropriate. The complexity is obvious, not to say marked, and it is often not possible to maintain experimental control without losing realism and dynamics. From a practical and applied point of view, it is desirable to assess experts in their natural, dynamic environment during, for example, training sessions or operational field exercises. From a researcher's point of view, it is usually not possible to interfere with (or actively manipulate) these environments; consequently, statistical methods have to be adjusted.

In studies of so-called natural situations, multivariate statistical analyses, based on covariation between variables, seem to be the most appropriate technique. As noted, these techniques explain to what extent treatments or training regimes have effects. As will be shown later, second generation multivariate techniques, such as SEM, make it possible to draw scientifically valid conclusions from studies of high realism and complexity.

Intra-Individual Variability and Repeated Measurement Designs

Most operational situations, like command and control environments, are dynamic and complex settings characterized by interacting and interdependent processes. In these situations, change and variability are distinctive characteristics of critical phases. As has been pointed out, change or variability can be seen as a transition from one, for the moment stable, state to another; the operator is considered as a dynamically changing human system (van Geert and van Dijk 2002). The variability of these processes is a function of preceding and current internal (psychological, physiological) and external (situational) conditions. Strictly, external conditions must be perceived and made internal in order to affect a human system. Previous events during a process can influence the current (as well as future) states of an operator. If, for example, information complexity has been high for a period, current workload may be increased and vigilance reduced. On the other hand, awareness of preceding arduous conditions may serve as a preparation for current and future similar situations by increasing mental effort. An operator can be seen as a self-regulating or self-organizing dynamic system (van Geert and van Dijk 2002). In the physical sciences, the study of dynamic systems has a long history.

Systematic variability is classified as an operator's response not only to the stimuli of the present situation but also to stimuli from previous situations; successive reactions more or less depend on preceding stimulus–response situations (Smith 1951; Fiske and Rice 1955). As will be shown, systematic intra-individual variability creates a base for systematic covariation, that is, the correlations between two or more time series variables.

Figure 4.1 illustrates the variation of two variables (variable A and variable B) as a function of situational changes over time (or phases) in a command and control mission. Vertical lines represent a series of phases. Horizontal broken lines represent participants' estimates of mental workload after each phase. Variable A represents system information load; variable B shows operator mental workload. One variable thus represents the dynamics of a technical system, whereas the other one visualizes the dynamics of an operator. The systems variable (A) is considered to be genuinely continuous, dynamic. Similarly, psychophysiological measures such as, for example, heart rate (an indirect measure of mental workload), as well as psychological or cognitive variables, are continuous. However, it is more difficult to measure the dynamics of cognitive variables such as workload, situational awareness and performance.

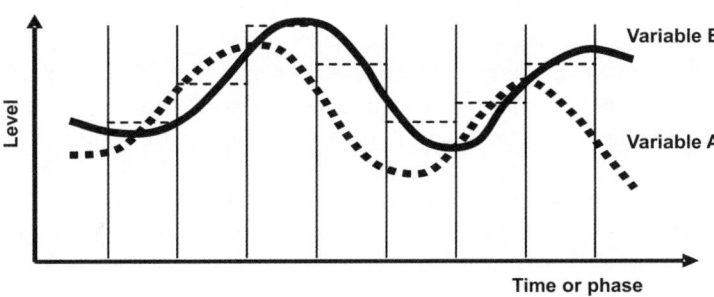

Figure 4.1   Variation of two variables (variable A: system information complexity; variable B: operator mental workload) over time in a command and control mission

In order to measure the psychological aspects as dynamically as possible, we use participants' repeated ratings of, for example, mental workload after certain time intervals or after work phases. These time series are discrete; they are estimates of continuous curves. The more often ratings or measures are made, the more detailed the estimations of the dynamics. Mental workload (B) in Figure 4.1 represents a discrete time series variable; the vertical lines indicate a series of phases representing natural work segments or time sequences. In the example, the participants were asked to repeatedly estimate their workload during the last phase. The horizontal broken lines in Figure 4.1 show the levels of the participants' estimates.

The simultaneous correlation between variables A and B in Figure 4.1 is .52, that is, the common variance is 27 per cent ($.52^2 = .27$). As can be seen, there appears to be a lag of about one phase between the variables, indicating that the operators' changes in workload (B) are delayed in relation to changes in the technical system's information load (A). If we correct this lag, the correlation increases to .87, that is, 76 per cent of the workload variance can be explained by the variance in systems information complexity. This type of cross-correlation between information load (A) and mental workload (B) illustrates how, for example, causal relations between time series variables can be estimated. Statistical assumptions concerning estimates of correlations between lagged variables (cross-correlations) are presented later.

Before presenting statistical techniques for time series analysis, we present (a) some characteristics of time series and (b) statistical assumptions that should be taken into consideration when performing time series analyses.

Types of Variation in Time Series

Time series variability can be argued to consist of four components: *trend*, *seasonal variability*, *other types of variability* and *irregular fluctuations*. Trend is a long-term change in the mean level. A long-term systematic change in performance as a function of training in command and control operations constitutes a trend component. Seasonal variability, next, represents periodic changes such as temperature or other (regular, predicted, expected and so on) weather fluctuations. In our case, variability in vigilance and human performance (as a result of circadian rhythms) forms a seasonal time series component since it involves regular repetition. So far, our experience from performance-related time series in command and control situations is that there are cyclic psychological changes as perceived information complexity, mental workload and situational awareness that differs over time and/or occasion. However, the regularity of the cycles changes as a function of non-cyclic situational influences. Changes in mental workload, for example, are most affected by a situation, to some extent by time of day, but not by time of year. This type of time series variability, thus, represents the so-called other types of variability. Having removed the variability from trend and different cyclic components, we find a series of random variations called irregular fluctuations. Such fluctuations are related to pure intra-individual variability or error variance (Chatfield 2004).

Stationarity in Time Series

A considerable part of probability theory, and the statistical assumptions of time series analysis, concerns and depends on stationary time series. In order to properly use time series analyses for modelling and forecasting, a non-stationary series needs to be transformed to a stationary series. A time series is argued to be stationary if there is no systematic change in mean and no trend over time; no systematic change in variance over time; and no systematic change in covariance between time series over time. Nevertheless, it is important to emphasize that a non-stationary component as the trend can be of more interest than stationary residuals (Chatfield 2004), which is the case for studies of, for example, training and skill retention effects (Svensson et al. 2013). In the examples given next, we remove trends to analyse local fluctuations, so-called other types of variability (for example workload and situational awareness) over time. The main reason why stationarity is required is that lagged auto- and cross-correlations are sensitive to, and can even be exaggerated by, trended time series.

Plotting and Smoothing Time Series

The first stage in time series analysis is to plot observations against time. From these plots, components such as trends, systematic and/or random fluctuations and discontinuities in variability can be detected. Time series can be more or less 'noisy' and might contain random and irregular variability. In these cases, it can be difficult to 'hear' (or see) through the noise and to discover the profile, or function, generating the series. By smoothing the series, the noise can be filtered and underlying functions easily seen. Smoothing is relatively easily carried out by *distance-weighted least squares regression* (DWLS), an efficient technique available in standard statistical packages (for example SPSS, Systat and Statistica). The resulting curves represent a 'running mean' determined by DWLS values. Unlike linear and polynomial smoothing, the surface is allowed to locally flex to fit data better. This flexibility can be chosen by a tension parameter (Wilkinson 1990a, 1990b). More flex implies that the curve will be closer to the data points, resulting in a 'noisier' curve. Less flex gives a smoother curve, but is not as close to the data. This smoothing technique also interpolates missing values. Figure 4.2 illustrates a time series plot of situational awareness ratings as a function of occasion. The discrete values are transformed into a curve or function by means of DWLS regression. The smoothed discrete values are estimations of the continuous variable situational awareness and can also be saved for further analysis.

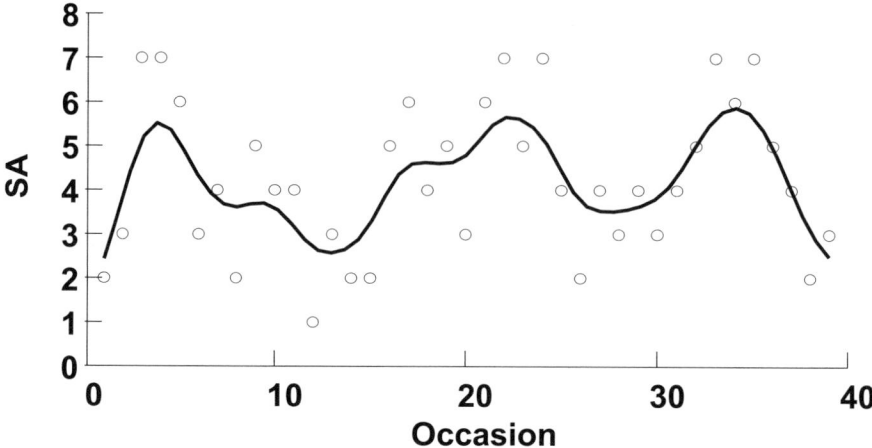

Figure 4.2   A time series plot of situational awareness (SA) as a function of situational changes over time

Autocorrelations

Autocorrelation coefficients measure the correlation between observations or measures at different times or lags apart and show the relation of each point in time to a previous point in time in a series. The autocorrelation at lag 0 represents the simultaneous correlation between the data column and itself and is always equal to 1.0. The autocorrelation at lag 1 represents the correlation between a data column and its copy moved down one time point. If the autocorrelations at lag 1 are high, then every value highly correlates with the value at the previous time point (Wilkinson 1996). Lagged correlations will be illustrated and used later in our example on DFA. Autocorrelation functions are important tools when modelling or fitting suitable models to observed time series. For example, autocorrelation plots or 'correlograms' are useful when attempting to identify the most appropriate type of *autoregressive integrated moving average* (ARIMA) model (Chatfield 2004).

Autocorrelation plots are important when analysing whether time series are stationary or not. As noted above, time series analysis techniques (such as modelling) are sensitive to non-stationary series; therefore these series have to be transformed into stationary series before using modelling and forecasting techniques.

Non-stationary time series in terms of trends are of specific interest in our case because they affect lagged cross-correlations. If, for example, two series are trended with increasing values, early values in both series are smaller; later values larger. This produces large and trend-dependent positive correlations that, as it were, die out slowly as a function of lag and shadow true correlations from short-term variations of the curves. Stationary series exhibit short-term

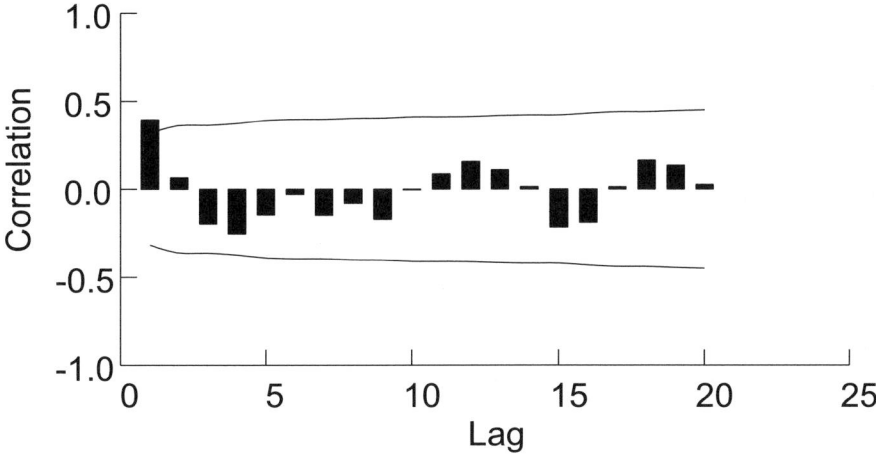

Figure 4.3   Autocorrelation plot. A correlogram showing the autocorrelation of the situational awareness variable in Figure 4.2

correlations characterized by large and significant coefficients for the first followed by one or two significant correlations (Chatfield 2004). Figure 4.3 shows the autocorrelation plot of the situation awareness variable in Figure 4.2. The plot shows the size of autocorrelations from lag 1 to lag 20. The columns indicate the size of the correlation at every lag. The lines mark the 95 per cent confidence level for the significance of every correlation. As can be seen from the plot, only the first autocorrelation is significant; accordingly, the series is stationary. Another conclusion is that every value correlates with the value at the previous time point of the series. The autocorrelation for lag 1 is .40, which means that 16 per cent of the variability of situational awareness at the second time point can be explained by the variability in the first.

Cross-correlations

Techniques such as modelling and forecasting are concerned with single time series. Apart from the illustration in Figure 4.1, we have hitherto discussed theoretical and statistical assumptions and techniques for analysing single time series. Next, we turn to situations where two or more time series are observed, being interested in their relationships. The correlation between two time series is of interest for two reasons, namely by forming *simultaneous relations* and *causal relations*. As an example, it can be important to analyse seismic signals from different sites because their simultaneous correlations need to be more fully explored. In addition to this (as in Figure 4.1), two time series might have interesting *causal relations* (Chatfield 2004). In Figure 4.1, a possible causal relationship between mental workload and information complexity was illustrated.

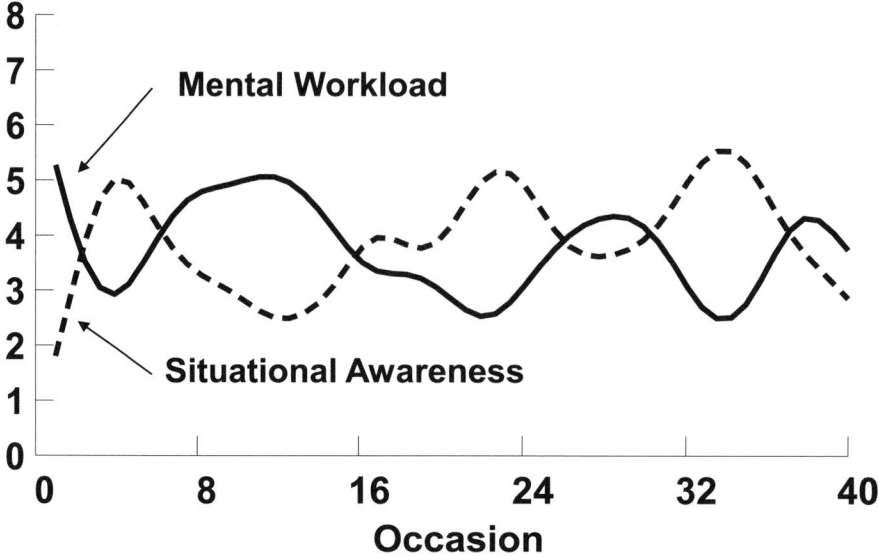

Figure 4.4   Time series plots of mental workload and situational awareness over time

As noted above, a trended time series inflates autocorrelations. In the same way, two trended time series inflate variances of cross-correlations. As for autocorrelations, a time series correlates with itself; regarding stationary series, there are no systematic changes over time in variance. Similarly, there are no systematic changes over time in covariance between two stationary cross-correlated series. Like the autocorrelation function, the cross-correlation function is an important tool for analyses and identification of variability, relations and time delays.

Figure 4.4 illustrates time series plots of mental workload and situational awareness as a function of occasion. The discrete values are transformed into curves or functions by means of DWLS regression. The situational awareness curve is the same as that in Figure 4.2. As can be seen, the curves are inverted; increases in mental workload relate to decreases in situational awareness.

The autocorrelation plot of the mental workload series was similar to the autocorrelation plot of the situation awareness series in Figure 4.3; accordingly, both series are stationary, have no trends. The stationarity of the series reduces the risk for trend-dependent correlations and increases the influence of local fluctuations on cross-correlations.

Figure 4.5 shows a cross-correlation plot of the series mental workload and situational awareness. The columns indicate the size of the correlation at every lag. The lines mark the 95 per cent confidence level for the significance of every correlation. The simultaneous correlation at lag 0 is -.77 ($p < .001$), that is, the

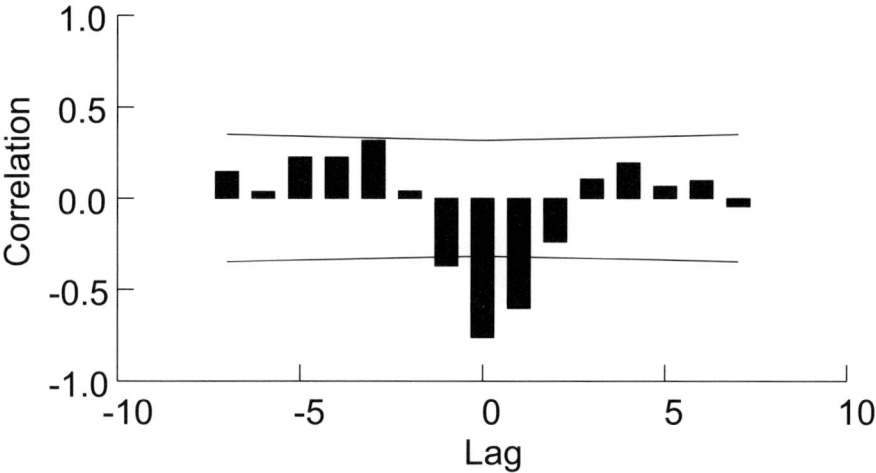

Figure 4.5   **Cross-correlation plot. A correlogram showing the cross-correlation of mental workload and situational awareness**

variability in mental workload explains 59 per cent of the simultaneous variability in situational awareness. However, it can be seen that there is a significant and high correlation of -.65 ($p < .001$) at lag 1. This means that the variability in mental workload explains 42 per cent of the variability in situational awareness one occasion later and mental workload can be seen as a prominent indicator or cause of later changes in situational awareness.

In the illustrations above, both time series (mental workload and situational awareness) were found to be stationary, and thus appropriate for most time series analysis techniques. However, time series are not *always* stationary, so how are trended time series to be handled? One answer to this question is that there are transformation procedures or filtering techniques that effectively remove trends and non-stationary variability of time series.

As was mentioned previously, we are particularly interested in lagged cross-correlations, more specifically the correlation between one variable and another variable at a later time in a series. Unfortunately, such correlations tend to be inflated by trended series. For this reason, transformations that 'de-trend' time series are essential. A transformation technique which is particularly useful for removing trends is that which *differences* time series. Through *difference*, thus, every value in a series is replaced by the difference between this and a previous value. This type of first-order differencing is widely used and removes trends effectively (Chatfield 2004). A way to remove non-stationary variability may be to replace the values in a series with their natural logarithms. To square the values in the series may normalize variance across the series (Wilkinson 1996). It is important to note that no information can be lost through these transformations; thus an original time series can be reconstructed from transformed values.

A general point of view on transformations is, however, that they should be used with judgement. Non-stationary components (such as trends) may sometimes be more interesting than stationary residuals (Chatfield 2004). The suggested transformations here are all available in standard statistical packages (such as SPSS, Systat and Statistica).

Data Reduction and Modelling of Time Series

Having discussed theoretical and statistical assumptions, as well as techniques for analysis of (a) single time series and (b) the relations between two time series, attention is now drawn to situations where observations on several time series are available. The next focus or interest is thus simultaneous and lagged relationships.

Figure 4.6 represents a general example of the variability of several systems and operator time series variables as a function of time (phases) during a command and control mission. The complexity is apparent and it is difficult to investigate the relationships even if the number of variables is relatively low. By means of data reduction techniques complexity can be managed, facilitating explanations and interpretations. By statistical modelling techniques causal relations between underlying dynamic dimensions can be demonstrated or confirmed. Dynamic modelling is a way of unfolding behaviour across time (Bertenthal 2007).

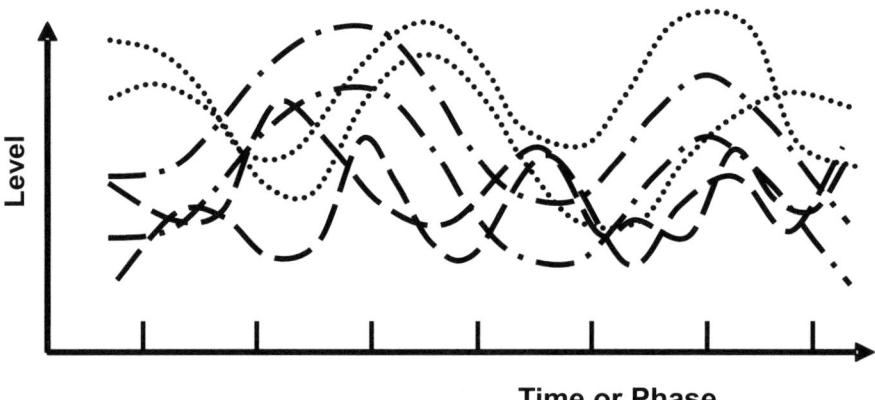

Time or Phase

Figure 4.6   **Variation of variables as a function of time in a simulated command and control mission**

Statistical Techniques

Factor analysis (FA) is an analytical technique that makes it possible to reduce a larger number of interrelated manifest variables to a smaller number of latent variables or factors. FA is based on the covariation between manifest measured variables; its aim is to produce a simplified description by using the smallest number of explanatory concepts required to explain the maximum amount of variable variation (the common variance in a correlation matrix). Factors that are generated by FA are a type of hypothetical construct, latent factors, explaining covariation between their markers. The constructs find their manifest expression in their markers (Hair et al. 1998).

Dynamic factor analysis (DFA) is a technique applicable to multivariate time series. Initial attempts to model intra-individual variability by means of the common factor model were carried out by Cattell (Cattell et al. 1947), and referred to as *P-factor analysis*. In contrast to classical factor analysis (which factors the inter-individual variance), DFA factors intra-individual variance. Accordingly, a main difference between classical analysis and DFA is found in the input matrix. Within classical factor analysis, the input matrix represents concurrent correlations between variables; in DFA it represents concurrent *and* lagged correlations between time series variables. In contrast to classical factor analysis, DFA can be performed on time series data from one or a few participants (Nesselroade and Molenaar 2004; Molenaar 2006). Due to its predictive potential, DFA has so far mostly been used within the economical sciences (Molenaar 2006). A recent example of psychological studies concerns validation of clinical and cognitive case formulations (Mumma and Mooney 2007); an older example is that of emotional response patterns underlying relationships in families (Hershberger et al. 1994).

In SEM, linear structural relationship and the factor structure are combined into one comprehensive model applicable to observational studies. The model allows (a) multiple latent constructs indicated by observable explanatory (or exogenous) variables, (b) recursive and non-recursive relationships between constructs and (c) multiple latent constructs indicated by observable response (or endogenous) variables. The connections between the latent constructs compose the structural equation model; the relationships between the latent constructs and their observable indicators or outcomes compose the factor model (Jöreskog and Sörbom 1993: xxiv). All parts of the comprehensive model can be represented in a path diagram; all factor loadings and structural relationships appear as coefficients of the path. A structural equation modelling technique called LISREL (*linear structural relationships*) gives a series of goodness of fit measures to the whole model (Jöreskog and Sörbom 1993; Hair et al. 1998).

Usually, a square, symmetric variance and covariance matrix based on inter-individual variability forms the input data for a SEM analysis; the statistical assumptions (such as independence of measures and number of cases) of the technique are based on this condition. However, the flexibility of the LISREL software concerning measurement errors, and restrictive assumptions, makes it particularly suitable for data reduction and modelling of repeated measures and time series data. When it comes to correlated measurement errors, it is reasonable to assume that the errors associated with observed or manifest variables correlate over time. Correlated errors may and ought to be included in the model estimation (Jöreskog and Sörbom 1993; Wood and Brown 1994). Other features that make SEM an ideal technique for modelling time series data are multiple markers (making latent variables reliable) and indirect paths (easily accommodated) (Little et al. 2006). The illustrations of DFA below are performed by means of SEM modelling, more specifically LISREL (Jöreskog and Sörbom 1993; Zhang and Browne 2010).

We have mentioned that discrete time series can, and often do, represent genuine continuous variables; repeated questions at an ordinal level of genuinely continuous psychological variables (for instance mental workload, situational awareness, performance) are examples of this. The general factor analytic model is adapted to correlations between underlying continuous manifest variables rather than to direct correlations between discrete and ordinal manifest variables. The most commonly used input matrix to factor analyses is based on *Pearson's product moment correlations*. This covariation measure can, however, render suboptimal estimates of underlying correlations between continuous variables. The *polychoric* correlation is a better alternative as it represents the 'true' correlation between underlying continuous variables. Factor loading estimates based on polychoric correlations are found to be less biased and often higher than loadings based on product moment correlations. Accordingly, factors based on polychoric correlations are expected to be more reliable. The polychoric coefficient is estimated from a contingency table formed by observations on the two ordinal manifest variables (Jöreskog and Sörbom 1996; Zhang and Browne 2010). By means of a preprocessor to LISREL (PRELIS), multivariate data screening and estimations of polychoric, as well as Pearson correlations, can be made (Jöreskog and Sörbom 1996).

Data reduction and modelling involving LISREL have been carried out since the 1980s in the human factors group at the Swedish Defence Research Agency (Totalförsvarets Forskningsinstitut, FOI). Examples relating to military and civil aviation are given in, for example, Svensson et al. (1993, 1997b), Svensson (1997), Svensson and Wilson (2002), Berggren (2000), Nählinder et al. (2004), Castor (2009) and Nählinder (2009). Within the framework of NATO research, studies on selection of command and control leaders, and personnel predictive modelling of personality traits, have been realized using LISREL (Svensson et al. 2008).

Because the input matrix to SEM programs must be square and symmetric, *Toeplitz transformation* is used. This method represents the simultaneous and lagged covariances across variables in a square and symmetric matrix. The transformation to a square and symmetric matrix is performed by duplicating the blocks of variances and covariances in a diagonal way (Wood and Brown 1994).

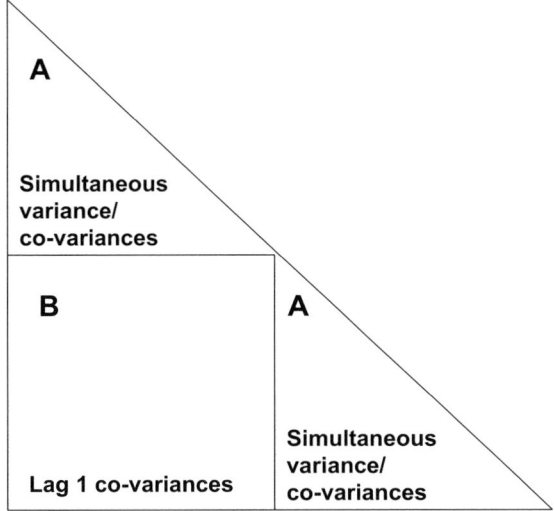

Figure 4.7   Toeplitz-transformed covariances for a window size of two replications

Figure 4.7 presents a graphic representation of a Toeplitz transformation in the case of a window size of two replications, and one lag.

First the simultaneous correlations (where lag = 0) between the time series variables were calculated. Then the time series were lagged one occasion (one time unit lag of measurement on themselves and on each other). This means that the variables are correlated with their own values as well as the values of the other variables on the occasion before.

To illustrate the DFA technique, a subset of data from a study at a Swedish Air Command Operations Centre (COC) is used. Officers operating the COC answered questions on mental workload (WL), information complexity (COMP), situational awareness (SA) and performance (PERFI) every tenth minute on *personal data assistant systems* (PDA) during a simulated command and control operation. Before the simultaneous and lagged correlations between the four time series variables were calculated, the assumptions of stationarity were controlled (see above: no systematic trends; constant variance of each variable over time; constant covariances between variables across occasions). The requirement of no trend was examined by regressions predicting the variables as a function of time. The other requirements were examined by ocular inspections of curves smoothed by means of DWLS. From regression analysis, a significant trend was found for workload, and, accordingly, the variable was de-trended. No other indications of non-stationarity could be identified.

Table 4.1 **Correlation matrix for mental workload (WL), information complexity (COMP), situational awareness (SA) and performance (PERFI) over time**

	WL	COMP	SA	PERFI
WL	1.00	–	–	–
COMP	0.72	1.00	–	–
SA	-0.25	-0.21	1.00	–
PERFI	-0.16	-0.15	0.69	1.00
WL1	*0.25*	0.26	-0.05	0.05
COMP1	0.27	*0.31*	-0.12	-0.01
SA1	-0.05	-0.06	*0.10*	0.04
PERFI1	-0.03	-0.03	0.05	*-0.02*
WL2	*0.22*	0.23	-0.01	0.01
COMP2	0.22	*0.23*	-0.01	0.03
SA2	-0.05	-0.08	*0.02*	0.06
PERFI2	-0.05	-0.02	-0.05	*-0.02*

In Table 4.1, the upper symmetric square matrix shows the simultaneous (lag 0) correlations. The second asymmetric square matrix (WL1–PERFI1) shows the correlations between the variables at the lag 1 occasion, and the third asymmetric square matrix the correlations at the lag 2 occasion. Diagonal values of the matrices (in italics) indicate autocorrelations, and off-diagonal values cross-correlations. In the final symmetric input matrix, the upper symmetric square matrix is replicated twice, and the second asymmetric square matrix is replicated once.

We start the analysis by modelling the simultaneous model using only the symmetric square matrix showing the simultaneous (lag 0) covariances between WL, COMP, SA and PERFI. Figure 4.8 illustrates the final 'simultaneous model'. The fit of the model is virtually perfect with a *mean square error of approximation* (RMSEA) = .000 and a *comparative fit index* (CFI) = .99. This means that the factors and the effect of the model fully explain the correlations of the input matrix. As can be seen, the four latent time series variables have been reduced to two factors referred to as mental workload (MWL) and performance (PERF). This factor structure represents the measurement model of the SEM analysis. The causal effect of -.28 between the mental workload and performance factors represents the structural model of the analysis. The general conclusion of the model is that performance decreases as a function of increases in mental workload.

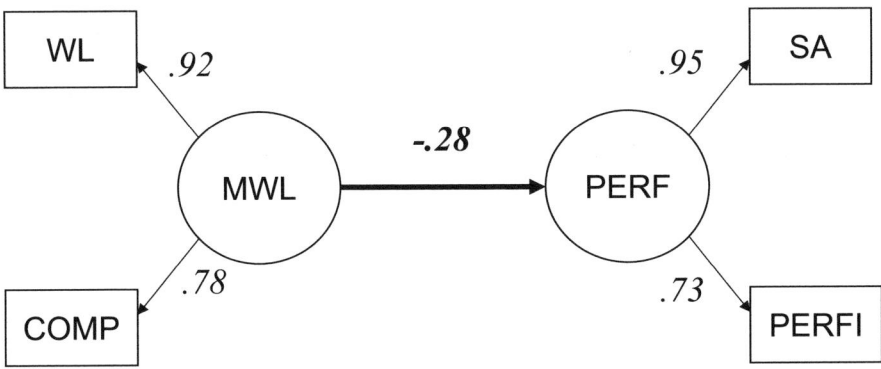

Figure 4.8   **Structural equation model based on simultaneous (lag = 0) correlations between variables mental workload (WL), information complexity (COMP), situational awareness (SA) and individual performance (PERFI)**

To continue, we analyse if, and to what extent, the factors in the simultaneous model (see Figure 4.8) are affected by their values 10 and 20 minutes before. Lag 1 represents the correlations 10 minutes before, and lag 2 the correlations 20 minutes before. A hypothesis is that both mental workload and performance affect their later conditions (they were set free in the analysis). Figure 4.9, presenting the final model, shows that only mental workload is affected by its conditions 10 and 20 minutes before.

The fit of the final dynamic model is high with an RMSEA = 0.023, a CFI = 0.99, an NFI = .97 and an NNFI = .99. The high fit means that the factors and effects of the model almost completely explain the correlations of the input matrix.

In the initial analysis of the dynamic model, the factors (mental workload and performance) were set free to influence later occasions. But, as can be seen in Figure 4.9, only workload influences later occasions to a significant extent. At any given occasion (as in Figure 4.8), mental workload has a negative effect on performance; if an operator has high mental workload, this affects his or her performance negatively. Apparently, only mental workload links occasions over time. This means that mental workload affects itself on later occasions, and there is a significant indirect effect of workload at the first time point on the third time point 20 minutes later. It is also found that mental workload at a certain time point has significant indirect effects on performance at a later point in time, specifically 10 and 20 minutes later. It is important to notice that performance at a certain point in time has no effect on performance at a later occasion; only mental workload affects performance at later points in time. It should also be observed that the dynamic model has a simplex structure, and that the change process of mental workload progresses at a constant linear rate over time (Little et al. 2006; Castor 2009).

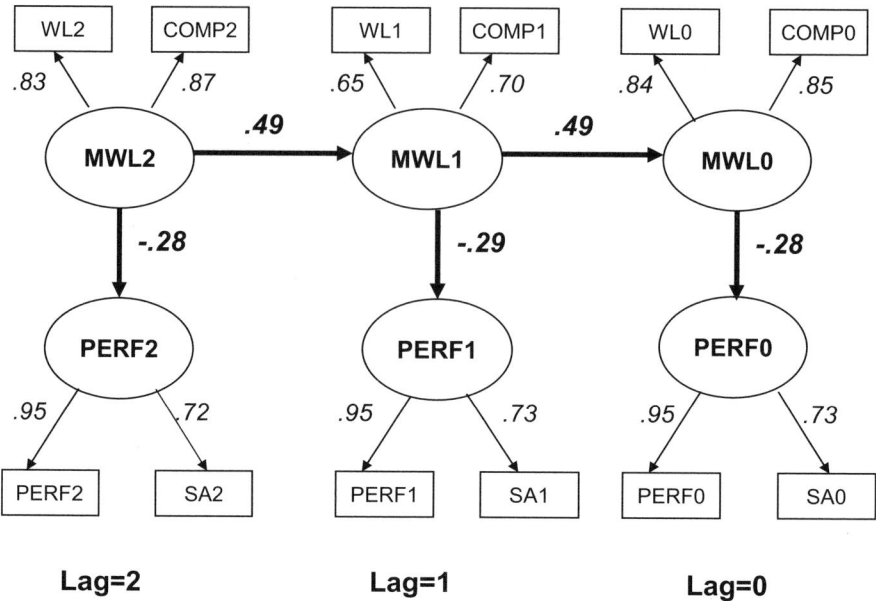

Figure 4.9   Final SEM model based on the simultaneous (lag = 0), the lag = 1 and the lag = 2 correlations between variables mental workload (WL), information complexity (COMP), situational awareness (SA) and individual performance (PERFI)

Conclusions

The command and control environment is a dynamic and complex setting with technical systems and operators, or teams of operators, interacting to reach shared goals. Classical experimentation designs and static measures are, in many respects, insufficient tools for dynamic situations, where designs and measures adapted to natural environments are needed. Accordingly, the focus needs to be on dynamic changes or processes over periods of time; process measures are called for. We have shown how to estimate so-called true relations (cross-correlations) between time series measures (that is, relations between dynamic changes of variables), and also how their ability to predict future events can be investigated. We have explained the importance of variance and change in experimentation and measurement, and the basic differences between inter- and intra-individual sources of variance. The components of repeated measures or time series (levels or mean value, long-term movements and seasonal – periodical – changes) have been elucidated. Statistical considerations such as stationarity with respect to systematic trends, variance constancy of variables and constancy of covariance over time of time series have been explained, as well as their importance for optimal estimates of covariation. Our conclusion is that systematic trends in particular have to be controlled because of their tendency to exaggerate auto- and cross-correlations. Important techniques for transformation and smoothing of time series have been demonstrated; transformations as de-trending of series result in more faultless estimates of correlation, and smoothing facilitates the finding and inspection of profiles and functions of time series. In the development and operational evaluation of command and control systems, important human factors aspects are mental workload (information load), situational awareness (situation assessment, understanding and attention) and performance (decision-making). Using these aspects, we demonstrated that dynamic factor analysis is an efficient statistical technique for analysis and reduction of a larger number of manifest time series variables into a smaller set of dynamic factors. The conclusions of our example were that increases in mental workload decrease performance, and, unlike performance, mental workload affects or predicts later workload and performance. Finally, we demonstrated that structural equation modelling involving LISREL is particularly suitable for dynamic factor analyses.

References

Angelborg-Thanderz, M. (1997). Military pilot performance: Dynamic decision-making in its extreme. In R. Flin, E. Salas, M. Strub and L. Martin (eds), *Decision Making Under Stress: Emerging Themes and Applications*. Aldershot: Ashgate, 225–32.

Berggren, P. (2000). *Situational Awareness, Mental Workload and Pilot Performance – Relationships and Conceptual Aspects.* FOA–R–00–01438–706–SE, ISSN 1104–9154.

Berggren, P. (2005). Observing situational awareness: When differences in opinion appear. In H. Montgomery, R. Lipshitz and B. Brehmer (eds), *How Professionals Make Decisions*. Mahwah, NJ: Lawrence Erlbaum Associates, 233–41.

Bertenthal, B.I. (2007). Dynamical systems: It's about time! In S.M. Boker and M.J. Wenger (eds), *Data Analytic Techniques for Dynamical Systems*. Mahwah, NJ: Lawrence Erlbaum Associates.

Boff, K.R. (2006). Revolutions and shifting paradigms in human factors and ergonomics. *Applied Ergonomics*, 37, 391–9.

Browne, M.W. and Zhang, G. (2007). Repeated time series models for learning data. In S.M. Boker and M.J. Wenger (eds), *Data Analytic Techniques for Dynamical Systems in the Social and Behavioral Sciences*. Mahwah, NJ: Lawrence Erlbaum Associates.

Caldwell, J.A., Wilson, G.F., Cetinguc, M., Gaillard, A.W.K., Gundel, A., Lagarde, D., Makeig, S., Myhre, G. and Wright, N.A. (1994). *Psychophysiological Assessment Methods*. AGARD–AR–324. Neuilly-sur-Seine, France: Advisory Group for Aerospace Research and Development.

Castor, M. (2009). *The Use of Structural Equation Modeling to Describe the Effect of Operator Functional State on Air-to-Air Engagement Outcomes*. Linköping Studies in Science and Technology. Dissertations; 1251. ISBN 978-91-7393-657-6.

Cattell, R.B., Cattell, A.K.S. and Rhymer, R.M. (1947). P-technique demonstrated in determining psychophysical source traits in a normal individual. *Psychometrica*, 12, 267–88.

Chatfield, C. (2004). *The Analysis of Time Series*. New York: Chapman & Hall/CRC.

Deboeck, P.R. and Boker, S.M. (2010). Unbiased, smoothing-corrected estimation of oscillators in psychology. In S.M. Chow, E. Ferrer and F. Hsieh (eds), *Statistical Methods for Modelling Human Dynamics: An Interdisciplinary Dialogue*. New York, London: Routledge, Taylor & Francis Group, 13–37.

Ferrer, E. and Nesselroade, J.R. (2003). Modeling affective processes in dyadic relations via dynamic factor analysis. *Emotion*, 3(4), 344–60.

Fiske, D.W. and Rice, L. (1955). Intra-individual response variability. *Psychological Bulletin*, 52(3), 217–50.

Hair, J.F., Jr., Anderson, R.E., Tatham, R.L. and Black, W.C. (1998). *Multivariate Data Analysis*. New Jersey: Prentice Hall.

Hershberger, S.L., Corneal, S.E. and Molenaar, P.C. (1994). Dynamic factor analysis: An application to emotional response patterns underlying daughter/father and stepdaughter/stepfather relationships. *Structural Equation Modeling*, 2(1), 31–52.

Jöreskog, K. and Sörbom, D. (1993). *LISREL: Structural Equation Modeling with the SIMPLIS Command Language*. Chicago: Scientific Software International Inc.

Jöreskog, K. and Sörbom, D. (1996). *PRELIS2: User's Reference Guide*. Chicago: Scientific Software International Inc.

Little, T.D., Bovaird, J.A. and Slegers, D.W. (2006). Methods for the analysis of change. In D.K. Mroczek and T.D. Little (eds), *Handbook of Personality Development*. New York: Lawrence Erlbaum Associates.

Molenaar, P.C.M. (2006). The future of dynamic factor analysis in psychology and biomedicine. *Bull. Soc. Sci. Med.*, 2, 201–13.

Molenaar, P.C.M. and Ram, N. (2010). Dynamic modeling and optimal control of intraindividual variation: A computational paradigm for nonergodic psychological processes. In S.M. Chow, E. Ferrer and F. Hsieh (eds), *Statistical Methods for Modelling Human Dynamics: An Interdisciplinary Dialogue*. New York, London: Routledge, Taylor & Francis Group.

Mumma, G.H. and Mooney, S.R. (2007). Comparing the validity of alternative cognitive case formulations: A latent variable, multivariate time series approach. *Cognitive Therapy and Research*, 31, 451–81.

Nesselroade, J.R. (1991). Interindividual differences in intraindividual changes. In J.L. Horn and L. Collins (eds), *Best Methods for the Analysis of Change*. Washington, DC: American Psychological Association.

Nesselroade, J.A. and Molenaar, P.C.M. (2004). Applying dynamic factor analysis in behavioural and social sciences research. In Kaplan, D. (ed.), *The Sage Handbook of Quantitative Methodology for the Social Sciences*. California: Sage Publications Inc.

Nählinder, N. (2009). *Flight Simulator Training: Assessing the Potential.* Linköping Studies in Science and Technology. Dissertation; 1250. ISBN 978-91-7393-658-3.

Nählinder, S., Berggren, P. and Svensson, E. (2004), Reoccurring LISREL patterns describing mental workload, situation awareness and performance. *Proceedings of the Human Factors and Ergonomics Society 48th Annual Meeting*. New Orleans, LA: Human Factors and Ergonomics Society.

Shifren, K., Hooker, K., Wood, P. and Nesselroade, J.R. (1997). Structure and variation of mood in individuals with Parkinson's disease: A dynamic factor analysis. *Psychology and Aging*, 12(2), 328–39.

Smith, B.B. (1951). On some difficulties encountered in the use of factorial designs and analysis of variance with psychological experiments. *British Journal of Psychology*, 42, 250–68.

Svensson, E. (1997). Pilot mental workload and situational awareness – psychological models of the pilot. In Flin, R., Salas, E., Strub, M. and Martin, L. (eds), *Decision Making Under Stress: Emerging Themes and Applications*. Aldershot: Ashgate.

Svensson, E., Angelborg Thanderz, M., Castor, M. and Borgvall, J. (2013). Skill decay, re-acquisition training, and transfer studies in the Swedish Air Force: A retrospective review. In Arthur, W., Day, E., Bennet, W. and Portrey, A. (eds), *Individual and Team Skill Decay: The Science and Implications for Practice*. New York: Routledge, Taylor and Francis Group.

Svensson, E., Angelborg-Thanderz, M. and Sjöberg, L. (1993). Mission challenge, mental workload and performance in military aviation, *Aviation, Space, and Environmental Medicine*, 64, 985–91.

Svensson, E., Angelborg-Thanderz, M., Sjöberg, L. and Olsson, S. (1997a). Information complexity: Mental workload and performance in combat aircraft, *Ergonomics*, 40, 362–80.

Svensson, E., Angelborg-Thanderz, M. and van Awermaete, J. (1997b). *Dynamic Measures of Pilot Mental Workload, Pilot Performance, and Situational Awareness*. Technical Report: VINTHEC–WP3–TR01. NLR: Amsterdam.

Svensson, E., Lindoff, J. and Sutton, J. (2008). Predictive modelling of personality traits – Implications for selection of operational personnel. *NATO HFM Symposium on Adaptability in Coalition Teamwork* (RTO–MP–HFM–142 TP/212). Copenhagen, Denmark: NATO Research and Technology Organisation.

Svensson, E., Rencrantz, C., Lindoff, J., Berggren, P. and Norlander, A. (2006). Dynamic measures for performance assessment in complex environments. *Proceedings of the 50th Annual Meeting of the Human Factors and Ergonomics Society*. San Francisco, CA: Human Factors and Ergonomics Society.

Svensson, E. and Wilson, G.F. (2002). Psychological and psychophysical models of pilot performance for systems development and mission evaluation, *The International Journal of Aviation Psychology*, 12(1), 95–110.

van Geert, P. and van Dijk, M. (2002). Focus on variability: New tools to study intra-individual variability in developmental data. *Infant Behaviour & Development*, 25, 340–74.

Wilkinson, L. (1990a). *SYSTAT: The System for Statistics*. Evanston, IL: Systat Inc.

Wilkinson, L. (1990b). *SYSTAT: The System for Graphics*. Evanston, IL: Systat Inc.

Wilkinson, L. (1996). *SYSTAT 6.0 for Windows: Statistics*. Chicago: SPSS Inc.

Wilson, G., Frazer, W., Beaumont, M., Grandt, M., Gundel, A., Varoneckas, G., Veltman, H., Svensson, E., Burow, A., Hockey, B., Edgar, E., Stone, H., Balkin, T., Gilliland, K., Schlegel, R.E. and van Orden, K. (2004). *Operator Functional State Assessment*. Neuilly-sur-Seine, France: NATO HFM–056/ TG–008.

Wood, P. and Brown, D. (1994). The study of intraindividual differences by means of dynamic factor analysis models: Implementation and interpretation. *Psychological Bulletin*, 116(1), 166–86.

Zhang, G. and Browne, M.W. (2010). Dynamic factor analysis with ordinal manifest variables. In S.M. Chow, E. Ferrer and F. Hsieh (eds), *Statistical Methods for Modelling Human Dynamics*. New York: Routledge, Taylor and Francis Group, 241–63.

Chapter 5

Organizational Agility – An Overview

B.J.E. Johansson and P.V. Pearce

Introduction

This chapter is intended as a record of emerging thoughts, drawing on relevant research material and pulling this material together to inform about ongoing discussions of what *agility* is and how this relates to command and control. The views expressed here are intended to be emerging sets of views that can be used to inform current and future research activities.

At the first NATO SAS-085 panel meeting (designated SAS-085#1; 15–18 March 2010, RTA Paris, C2 Agility and Requisite Maturity), members proposed a number of different views concerning agility and so-called *C2 agility*, including early thoughts on how it may be modelled. This chapter provides a developing perspective on some of the discussions; more specifically, on what could constitute agility, and what agility may mean in a military command and control setting.

Theory

In one of the first definitions of agility in the command and control context, proposed by Alberts and Hayes (2003), agility comprises six dimensions: *robustness*, *resilience*, *responsiveness*, *flexibility*, *innovation* and *adaptation*. According to our interpretation, some of these concepts overlap. Resilience, for example, is normally considered to comprise at least responsiveness and flexibility, and in some cases it could be argued that it includes robustness, although that relation possibly goes both ways. Collapsing responsiveness, flexibility and robustness into resilience means it is possible to reduce the dimensions of Alberts and Hayes (2003) into three: resilience, innovation and adaptation.

Within the field of resilience engineering, discussions similar to those in SAS-085#1 have taken place for many years. McDonald (2006) proposes a definition of resilience that in many respects catches the key properties of an agile system. In agreement with the idea of requisite variety, McDonald states that a system must be able to manage variability presented by the environment (McDonald 2006):

> If resilience is a system property, then it probably needs to be seen as an aspect of the relationship between a particular socio-technical system and the environment of that system. Resilience appears to convey the properties of being adapted to the requirements of the environment, or otherwise being able to manage the variability or challenging circumstances the environment throws up. [p. 156]

Being resilient is thus very close to being agile, although resilience focuses mostly on reactive behaviour. If an organization is to be considered as agile, it must be resilient, but also have the capability of foreseeing changes in the environment as well as in itself, that is, exhibiting acuity. Holsapple and Li (2008) proposed a similar definition in their review of previous research on agility:

> Agility is the result of integrating alertness to changes (recognizing opportunities/ challenges) – both internal and environmental – with a capability to use resources in responding (proactive/reactive) to such changes, all in a timely, flexible, affordable, relevant manner. [p. 6]

Within this definition Holsapple and Li (2008) identify the importance of awareness but suggest that agility can be both proactive and reactive. Interestingly, Holsapple and Li (2008) do not explicitly consider adaptability within this definition, but there is a suggestion that it could be implicit in the need to change following recognition of opportunities and challenges.

The dimensions of agility as they currently stand do not consider alertness/ awareness/acuity as a dimension and as such they could be interpreted as adopting a largely reactive stance when considering agility, that is, given an organization has been subjected to some effect, how does it react and how is it impacted by the application of the effect? For example, consider an organization's command and control network being attacked so that a physical effect is seen within the system. Using these dimensions it might be possible to consider how resilient and robust the organization has been given the attack, and what impact the attack has had on its survivability. The organization will consider the kinds of responses it can deliver, and the flexibility it has in delivering any response. Finally, it will be reflexive to the extent that it can learn from the events and adapt itself accordingly – in line with the concept of double-loop learning as presented by Argyris (1977). In this sense, the dimensions convey a sense of surviving an initial shock and also reacting to that shock through adaptation. Awareness and alertness are, however, terms that are hard to translate into real-world, observable/measurable entities. In concrete terms, an organization must be able to detect variability that may lead to unwanted consequences and to provide adequate counteractions. Effective monitoring and detection of deviations from a desired state is therefore a precondition for response. The monitoring/detection, in turn, depends on whether it is possible to define what the desired target state of the system is and whether appropriate indicators of this state and criteria for deviations can be found.

Military endeavours almost always take place in 'wild' environments, meaning environments that present a large degree of uncertainty, both internally in terms of military goals as well as in terms of the context. A typical contemporary military mission comprises fuzzy goals such as 'establishing peace' as well as a diverse set of antagonists, non-governmental organizations and coalition partners. In wild systems, the desired target state therefore depends heavily on the organization's ability to understand itself and its surroundings, as well as on the ability to articulate this in terms of appropriate actions (Johansson et al. 2002). A dichotomy can be sensed in the context of military agility, as a military system is designed with the intent of being highly structured and controllable, while at the same time acting in an environment that is characterized by the opposite conditions. The situation to be controlled is generally highly complex and depends on such a large number of factors that performance often is difficult to both predict and control. An important characteristic of a 'wild' system is that there is limited time available for 'getting to know' the 'system' to be controlled. The commanders' understanding, therefore, greatly depends on what they already know – their existing 'model' of the system and situation at hand – as well as on other articulated descriptions. The dissemination of adequate descriptions of the desired target state, such as commander's intent, is therefore a crucial determinant of how well a system is able to control a process (Builder et al. 1999). The ability to successfully disseminate a desired target state within an organization is also an important prerequisite for detection, and thus alertness, as it is only possible to detect and respond to changes in relation to something. As Charles S. Peirce said in 1868, 'every cognition is based on a previous cognition'.

At the same time, in order for an organization to observe changes it must have the appropriate 'eyes' in terms of the sensors and monitoring equipment needed to detect changes. This does not mean that the 'desired state' must be stated precisely. Conversely, the manifestation may be a very short order, supported by implicit understanding based on cultural, personal and organizational expectations, as well as knowledge about the current context and situation (Clark 1996; McCann and Pigeau 2000).

A proactive view of command and control agility should therefore explicitly include acuity as that is the basis for formulating the goals and states to be strived for. McDaniel et al. (2007) define four attributes of an agile organization, namely *awareness*, *flexibility*, *adaptability* and *productivity*. Importantly, McDaniel et al. (2007) pick up on acuity or the anticipatory element by suggesting that awareness is all about proactive sensing and proactive data gathering but, unlike Holsapple and Li (2008), the notion of adaptability is introduced.

McDaniel et al. (2007) use the term 'flexibility' to refer to appropriate responses to *expected* changes. 'Adaptability' is defined by McDaniel et al. (2007) as the ability of the organization to respond to unexpected events and add options accordingly. This is a different interpretation to that of Dyer and Shafer (1998), who defined organizational agility as *the capacity to be infinitely adaptable without having to change*, although arguably this is paradoxical as adaptation implies that change is required or has occurred. 'Productivity' is defined by Plummer and McCoy (2006) as the capacity to respond effectively while making efficient use of resources, but recognizing that these changes may be substantial and require innovation, involve risk and potentially be disruptive.

The proactive and reactive nature of agility is analogous to a social psychological theme called the agency–structure dualism, where agency theorizes that individuals, or in this case organizations, are agents of their own destiny free from the constraints of structure (process constraints and so on that may stop an organization exhibiting agency). Within this agency–structure dualism, it can be posited that acuity and flexible responses to detected threats would be analogous to agency, whereas structure would be analogous to back office functions that facilitate organizational adaptation and improve the range of options for a flexible response in future. Agility would therefore involve maintaining an appropriate balance between agency and structure for an organization to be effective. Dyer and Schafer (1998) give an example of this agency–structure dualism by referring to the term *chaordic*. Dyer and Shafer (1998) cite Dee Hock, former president of Visa International, who used the term to describe the need for organizations to be both chaotic and ordered to ensure agility, where chaos allows for initiative and innovation to flourish whilst doing something against a backdrop of systems that support overall coordination and cooperation. This can be viewed as a grid, as shown in Figure 5.1.

The act of balancing chaos and order in an organization is the challenge for anyone trying to design for agility. While providing the necessary structure for work, organization members must still be given freedom to be creative and take advantage of opportunities as they appear. Dyer and Shafer (1998) discuss two ways in which organizational performance can be improved to support this *chaordic* concept. One method, called adaptive or single-loop learning (Morgan 1997; Senge 1990), is analogous to the reflexive dimension of command and control agility put forward by the Focus, Agility and Convergence Team (a forum for command and control practitioners, theorists and analysts) and involves learning on a continuous basis to enable improvement to be made to the organization.

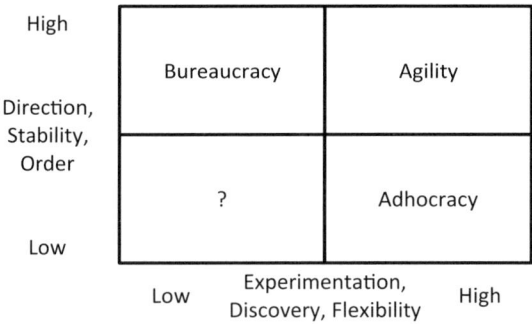

Figure 5.1   Agility as chaos and order, as in Dyer and Shafer (1998)

The second type of learning is referred to as generative or double-loop learning, based on the ideas of Argyris (1977, 1985). Dyer and Shafer (1998) state that this involves developing people and encouraging a culture within which people form new mental models of the external world and challenge the fundamental ethos and ways of working within the organization to enable different views of the external world to be considered. The 'norm' of such an organization is thus to constantly question current ways of working and seek new ways to cope with threats and take advantage of opportunities. Kjellén (1987) describes norms as something existing on *all* levels in an organization, ranging from the technical solutions at hand to management policies. Kontogiannis (2010) writes that reframing constructs and balancing stances from different team members may question the steering goals and eventually create strategies for replanning. This concept of generative learning maps onto the notion of developing a sense of awareness or acuity about the external environment to enable agility. Double-loop learning can therefore partly explain how an organization can change without having been subject to an external intervention, while single-loop learning only explains learning from experience. Interestingly, Dyer and Shafer (1998) discuss agile organizations as being self-organizing organizations, with self-organization centred on agile people, reconfigurable business processes, infrastructure and organizational designs. The concept of self-synchronizing organizations is very similar to the notion of the *edge command and control approach*, where the objective of edge command and control is to enable the collective to self-synchronize (NATO 2009).

One of the difficulties with the views on adaptation in previous research is that, from an evolutionary perspective, adaptation in response to environmental changes is a slow process, but within agility research the concept of adaptation becomes associated with notions of quickness, speed of thought and so on. One way of perhaps resolving this dichotomy is to think of adaptation from a slower evolutionary perspective. For example, organizations exhibit adaptation when they evolve new properties; original functions or capabilities are added to improve the overall fitness of the organization. This would place adaptation within a learning space. If adaptation can be viewed accordingly, then it is possible to bind organizational agility in terms of an awareness space covering acuity, that is, the ability to anticipate or to be aware and detect a change in the environment; a resilience space, where an organization can act and deliver an effect against a threat from a range of options and where the organization has a degree of shock absorption where a response fails to some extent; and a learning space within which adaptations take place and increase the range of response options. Gehler (2005) supports this notion and proposes a separation between awareness and learning, arguing that agility is a metaphor for awareness and adaptation a metaphor for learning. The separation of awareness is similar to a view put forward by Dekker (2006), who expands the traditional observe, orient, decide, act (OODA) loop and essentially phrases agility in terms that map onto acuity and having a range of options that can be considered in delivering an effect. This bounded awareness space is also analogous to the *adaptive action level* of Spaans et al. (2009).

Dekker (2006) also introduces the idea that agility requires capability strength *and* capability depth; strength referring to the size of a capability and depth to the duration for which that capability or response can be sustained. Both of these capabilities are similar to the notion of productivity (Plummer and McCoy 2006). The range of flexible options that an organization can consider in response to a threat is comparable to the notion of requisite variety within organizations (Dyer and Shafer 1998), enabling an organization to respond with appropriate action and deliver effects using the existing variety of capabilities against an expected or unexpected threat. At the SAS-085#1 meeting, the notion of manifest agility versus latent agility was discussed. By viewing flexibility of response as a dimension, it could be argued that manifest agility resides in the range of options that an organization has to deliver effects. The available time to choose an action is naturally an important constraint. If the time available is limited, it is very likely that the most obvious action will be chosen based on previous experience of similar situations, although that particular action may not be the best option. Lindblom (1959) labels this *muddling through*, an idea that is supported by more recent findings in, for example, *naturalistic decision-making* (Klein et al. 1993) or the *efficiency–thoroughness trade-off* (ETTO; Hollnagel 2009). Also, in a command and control situation, the spatial deployment of resources constrains what is possible and what is not. The manifest agility may thus differ between situations, depending on the temporal–spatial preconditions.

Where an organization fails to deal with a threat through one of its available responses, it can be argued that it does not have sufficient requisite variety among its people, processes, structures or infrastructure to be sufficiently productive to deliver action and effect within time. Should an organization not have sufficient requisite variety to deal with a threat (either a manifest threat or possible threat), *robustness* becomes important in determining the degree of shock absorption that an organization can take, for example an organization falls back onto its existing barriers and defences. Having a degree of shock absorption for risk mitigation may, however, require that the organization has an element of redundancy within its processes and systems. The ability to absorb shock and ensure a degree of robustness ensures that the organization can move to the learning space within which the organization considers its response to the threat, adapts its responses and increases its flexibility for dealing with threats of this type in the future. This adds yet another dimension to the balancing game – it is not enough to balance chaos and order, as suggested by Dyer and Schaefer (1998); there must also be a balance between the amount of resources spent on learning/adaptation and coping with current activities. This is analogous to the concept of capacity building in a business organization. Capacity building comes at the cost of production, but is necessary to survive in the long run. It is also essential to train and educate the personnel of a company if they are to recognize future trends and opportunities.

Conceptualizing agility in this way would suggest that time should be considered differently in the awareness and resilience spaces when compared to the learning space. If the organization is responding to a threat through delivery of existing flexible responses it is conceivable that the time to deliver a response would be different from the time to deliver a response if the organization has to rely on learning and adaptation to deliver options that enhance its flexibility and therefore enable delivery of a new effect. It is conceivable that an organization that has the necessary acuity can successfully anticipate or be aware of possible threats and therefore may recognize that it does not have the manifest agility to respond to a threat but it may have sufficient warning to enhance its flexibility prior to any threat being realized. Similarly, a response to anticipating threats may be to take proactive action to affect the environment; that is, risk mitigation activities.

Results

A synthesis of the ideas from previous research and the discussion above is made in Figure 5.2, which shows that a conceptual model of agility lies within an organization encompassing the system design/learning space put forward by Spaans et al. (2009). Essentially, one aspect of agility within this model sees the organization as being within a sense-and-respond loop (Dekker 2006; McDaniel et al. 2007), only breaking out of the loop when not able to offer an appropriate action to a manifest or possible threat. Experimentation, discovery and innovation would form part of the productivity input drawing on appropriate resources, skills and capabilities and considering capability size and depth (Dekker 2006). Learning takes place within the system design/learning space with reactive and proactive responses feeding into a continual learning activity challenging the organization to consider impacts on the resilience space. Within this conceptual model agility now encompasses five dimensions, those of *acuity, resilience, innovation, reflexivity* and *adaptation*.

There are now very different preconditions for proactive and reactive behaviour of a command and control organization. While the proactive dimension can be supported by encouraging (and providing time for) reflection and alternative thinking, the reactive dimension can be improved by supporting monitoring, detection and flexibility in response. Some case examples illustrate the concept below.

Consider, for example, a computer virus attack. An organization may already have anticipated some typical virus attack threats that are manifest in the environment and developed a number of options – or have the resilience (flexibility) – when meeting a threat. Upon detection of a threat, action would be taken drawing on options to meet the threat to deliver an effect back into the environment. This would have stayed within the agility space. Consider another manifest threat for which the organization has no options or lacks options to deal with the threat adequately. In this case, the threat penetrates the defences of the organization and so it falls back onto its manifest resilience (robustness) and the organization considers the impact on its survivability, that is, the damage it has suffered.

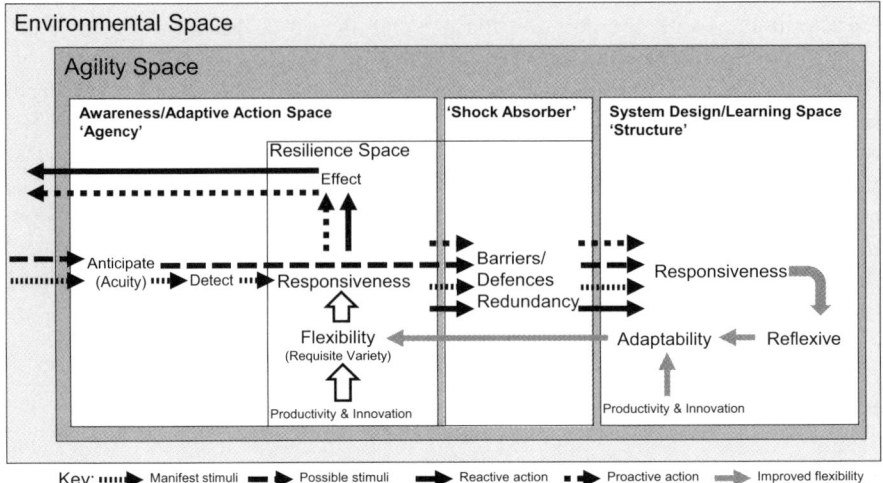

Figure 5.2   A conceptual view of agility

In time the organization responds by reflecting on the attack and considering how to adapt to the new threat. Reflection will involve the organization considering how it can increase its resilience, perhaps by considering a balance of investment between flexibility and robustness, each of which will have implications for overall organizational design. Similarly, potential threats could be anticipated for which there is no option for protecting against, and in this scenario the organization would again consider the impact of this threat materializing on its resilience (robustness) and would take a risk-based approach, considering responding and adapting to make new options available in case of attack. This corresponds to risk mitigation. In both cases eventual responses to the threat are fed into the system design space to facilitate continual learning.

Consider a network failure, where the threat may have been a risk related to systems reliability. Upon detection of the failure the organization would consider the options available, perhaps rerouting traffic and delivering an effect that maintains a network, although possibly having reduced throughput, back into the environment. Delivering action and effects from its resilient (flexible) store of options demonstrates agility. Not having options available would require the organization to take the 'shock' of the delivered effect and consider new capability and hence adaptation to deliver a new response option to mitigate against future failures. Again, in this case eventual responses to the threat are fed into the system design space to facilitate continual learning.

Conclusions

On the basis of previous research it is clear that there are a number of different perspectives on agility. Given these different perspectives on what constitutes agility and how the possible dimensions relate or not, the evidence to date suggests that agility is tangible and that it is something that organizations should aspire to. However, these different views on agility have put forward their own terms and definitions which are not always consistent. Despite these inconsistencies there are some common themes that can be drawn out. First, there is a theme concerning awareness or the ability to anticipate some effect on an organization, being proactive; secondly there is a theme regarding resilience and delivery of an appropriate response from a range of available response options, being reactive; thirdly there is a theme that emphasizes continual organizational learning, which is also synonymous with being reflexive and adaptable; fourthly there is arguably a theme concerning failure of an organization to respond effectively and thereby being able to absorb shock from an unexpected stimulus.

Distilling these themes we propose that agility can be considered as comprising five dimensions, namely acuity, resilience, reflexivity, adaptability and innovation. Further research should aim to concisely define these dimensions of agility, ensure that there is no ambiguity in their use and consider where the balance of agility fits within the agility space. How should the balance of investment be made across the agility space? The challenge will be to find an appropriate balance between chaos (freedom of action) and order (organizational control), as well as a balance between proactive and reactive capacity. This naturally depends on the context in which an organization is intended to operate, as different contexts demand different levels of agility. Ultimately, agility comes at the cost of control, but if future military forces are to be able to cope with the variety of contexts they will face, that sacrifice must be made.

References

Alberts, D.S. and Hayes, R.E. (2003). *Power to the Edge: Command, Control in the Information Age*. Washington, US: CCRP Publication Series.

Argyris, C. (1977). Organisational learning and management in information systems. *Accounting, Organizations and Society*, 2(2), 113–23.

Argyris, C. (1985). *Strategy, Change and Defensive Routines*. Boston, MA: Pitman.

Builder, C.H., Banks, S.C. and Nordin, R. (1999). *Command Concepts. A Theory Derived from the Practice of Command and Control*. RAND report.

Clark, H.H. (1996). *Using Language*. Cambridge: Cambridge University Press.

Dekker, A.H. (2006). Measuring the agility of networked military forces. *Journal of Battlefield Technology*, 9(1), 19–24.

Dyer, L. and Shafer, R.A. (1998). *From Human Resource Strategy to Organizational Effectiveness: Lessons from Research on Organizational Agility.* Centre for Advanced Human Resource Studies, Working Paper 98-12.

Gehler, C.P. (2005). *Agile Leaders, Agile Institutions: Educating Adaptive and Innovative Leaders for Today and Tomorrow.* Strategic Studies Institute. Available at http://www.strategicstudiesinstitute.army.mil/pubs/display. cfm?pubid=618 [accessed 10 February 2014].

Hollnagel, E. (2009). *The ETTO Principle: Efficiency–Thoroughness Trade-off.* Aldershot, UK: Ashgate Publishing Ltd.

Holsapple, C.W. and Li, X. (2008). Understanding organizational agility: A work–design perspective. *Proceedings of the 13th ICCRTS, Seattle, US*, 17–19 June 2008. Available at http://www.dodccrp.org/events/13th_ iccrts_2008/CD/Launch_CD.html [accessed 10 February 2014].

Johansson, B., Hollnagel, E. and Granlund, Å. (2002). The control of unpredictable systems. In C.W. Johnsson (ed.), *Proceedings of EAM2001.* GIST Technical Report G2002-1. Glasgow: University of Glasgow, 198–205.

Kjellén, U. (1987). Deviation and the feedback control of accidents. In J. Rasmussen, K. Duncan and J. Leplat (eds), *New Technology and Human Error.* Chichester: John Wiley & Sons Ltd, 143–53.

Klein, G., Orasanu, J., Calderwood, R. and Zsambok, E. (1993). *Decision-making in Action: Models and Methods.* Norwood, NJ: Ablex Publishing Corporation.

Kontogiannis, T. (2010). Adapting plans in progress in distributed supervisory work: Aspects of complexity, coupling and control. *Cognition, Technology & Work*, 12, 103–18.

Lindblom, C.E. (1959). The science of 'muddling through'. *Public Administration Quarterly*, 19, 79–88.

McCann, C. and Pigeau, R. (2000). The human in command. In C. McCann and R. Pigeau (eds), *The Human in Command: Exploring the Modern Military Experience.* New York: Kluwer Academic/Plenum Publishers, 1–9.

McDaniel, E., McCully, M. and Childs, R.D. (2007). Becoming a 'sense-and-respond' academic and government organisation. *The Electronic Journal of Knowledge Management*, 5(2), 215–22.

McDonald, N. (2006). Organizational resilience and industrial risk. In E. Hollnagel, D.D. Woods and N. Leveson (eds), *Resilience Engineering: Concepts and Precepts.* Aldershot: Ashgate Publishing Ltd, 155–79.

Morgan, G. (1997). *Images of Organizations.* 2nd ed. Thousand Oaks, CA: Sage.

NATO (2009). *NATO NEC C2 MATURITY MODEL*, SAS-065. Available at http://www.dodccrp.org [accessed 10 February 2014].

Plummer, D.C. and McCoy, D.W. (2006). *Achieving Agility: The View Through a Conceptual Framework.* Garter Research ID Number G00137820, 21 April 2006, as cited in McDaniel et al. (2007).

Senge, P.M. (1990). *The Fifth Discipline: The Art and Practice of the Learning Prganization.* New York: Doubleday.

Spaans, M., Spoelstra, M., Douze, E., Pieneman, R. and Grisogono, A.M. (2009). Learning to be adaptive. In *Proceedings of the 14th ICCRTS*, Washington DC, US, 15–17 June 2009. Available at http://www.dodccrp.org/events/14th_ iccrts_2009/Launch_CD.html [accessed 10 February 2014].

Chapter 6

Characteristics of Command and Control in Response to Emergencies and Disasters

J. Trnka and R. Woltjer

Introduction

The purpose of this chapter is to discuss the different aspects of command and control work in emergency and disaster response operations.

Response operations take place shortly after emergencies and disasters have occurred. They are carried out to save lives and to protect properties and the environment. They contain multiple goal-oriented activities aiming to mitigate the harmful consequences of emergencies and disasters.

A challenging aspect of emergencies and disasters is their dynamic and complex nature. They are characterized by a low degree of predictability of their magnitude and rate of change, as well as the temporal characteristics of this change. It can therefore be difficult to anticipate whether emergencies and disasters will escalate or suddenly change their nature, as well as when – and how fast – this change will take place. The dynamics and complexity of emergencies and disasters have implications for the way response operations are organized and the related command and control work conducted.

This chapter identifies the main characteristics of different types of response operations and their implications for command and control. The focus is thereby on the need-based character of emergency and disaster response operations, as well as the need for adaptations of the responding actors and their command and control structures. Key differences and commonalities in command and control between military operations and emergency and disaster response operations are identified, as well as their implications for joint operations.

Method

This chapter is a theoretical chapter. It discusses command and control in emergency and disaster response operations based on three presented key viewpoints. These viewpoints are grounded in different scientific concepts that are currently used in the domain of command and control in emergency and disaster response. The viewpoints are used to describe the main characteristics of present response operations supported by academic and practitioner literature and the authors' practical experience.

Results

This chapter identifies the main characteristics of emergency and disaster response operations. Our analysis is founded on three key viewpoints that we use to describe and discuss the main characteristics of response operations and the related command and control work. First, emergencies and disasters are distinctive phenomena that require specific management of response operations. Secondly, management of this type of response operation is a dynamic control process controlled by controllers. Thirdly, controllers need to be adaptive in multiple dimensions due to the nature of response operations.

Emergencies and Disasters are Distinctive Phenomena

The first key viewpoint is the view of emergencies and disasters as distinctive phenomena that require specific management of response operations. Emergencies, disasters and catastrophes are characterized by the existence of some sort of relatively unexpected threat that requires urgent action (Quarantelli 1993) or a negative, decisive turning point (Fredholm 2010). They are – in order of increasing severity in negative social consequences – quantitatively and qualitatively different phenomena, requiring different kinds of management (Quarantelli 2000, 2003).

Emergencies are situations where procedures, routines or plans are applicable to a large extent, including associated performance standards, but operational and command and control resources may be scarce. Organizations that need to cooperate to resolve a specific emergency are usually relatively familiar with working with each other, and their independence and interdependencies do not require major adaptations. Distinctions in responsibility between public and private sector are thus relatively clear. Most of the societal infrastructure is intact and victims can be taken care of by already existing societal resources, for instance community services and existing social structures, for example relatives (ibid.).

Disasters require large numbers of personnel from various organizations, often unfamiliar to each other and to working together. This may necessitate the emergence of new interdependencies among personnel and organizations and the loss of their independence. It may also result in new performance standards and often vague organizational (including public–private) responsibilities. The operational and command and control resources to deal with the disaster as well as the societal services in the disaster area are, however, largely intact, although some additional operational and command and control resources from other geographical areas may be required (ibid.).

Catastrophes are situations where most of the societal services, infrastructure as well as operational and command and control resources are unavailable and usual roles, plans, skills and responsibilities are not applicable, for a longer period of time. Resources and services from far outside the affected area need to be called in. Furthermore, normally existing social structures, like people getting help from relatives, cannot be relied on, due to the large-scale social effects of the societal crisis (ibid).

The triggers for these phenomena can be similar, such as natural events (for instance earthquakes, flooding, landslides), social friction (for instance social unrest), or industrial and transportation accidents. For the management of these events it is, however, their impact on society that is central. The impact may be characterized along several dimensions, for instance by the part and proportion of society that is affected and its geographical distribution; the onset, duration and recurrence. Examples of other dimensions are familiarity, predictability and severity of the impact of the event on the community or population; and the degree of preparedness and operational resource availability for the management of the response efforts (Quarantelli 1993).

The unique contexts and varying circumstances of emergencies, disasters and catastrophes therefore have an impact on how response operations are organized, how the related command and control work is conducted, as well as how collaborative work and interactions among personnel and organizations emerge. Response operations are governed by actual needs that are generated specifically by individual emergencies, disasters and catastrophes and can therefore be unique in their setup from event to event. From this perspective response operations are non-routine activities that require situation-driven and problem-solving management and behaviour by responding organizations and personnel (see, for instance, Comfort et al. 2001; Drabek and McEntire 2003; Kendra and Wachtendorf 2006).

In this chapter, we focus specifically on emergencies and disasters with a relatively sudden onset, which are usually handled at the local, regional or national emergency management level. Some emergency and disaster response characteristics may also be applicable to catastrophes (Quarantelli 2000), but by means of the sheer magnitude of their effects, often long-term international response as well as specific coordination and self-synchronization means (see, for example, Davidson et al. 1996; McEntire 1999; Suparamaniam and Dekker 2003; Hicks and Pappas 2006), catastrophes are beyond the explicit scope of this chapter.

Response Operations as a Dynamic Control Process

The second key viewpoint is founded in management of emergency and disaster response operations described as a dynamic control process. According to this viewpoint, emergency and disaster response operations are managed by controllers. These controllers are represented by socio-technical systems, consisting of people who use diverse artefacts, and whose activities are interrelated. The foundations of this viewpoint are the notion of dynamic control (see, for example, Brehmer and Allard 1991; Brehmer 1992), the basic cyclic model of control (Neisser 1976; Hollnagel 1998), cybernetic systems (Wiener 1948; Ashby 1956) and joint cognitive systems (Hollnagel and Woods 2005; Woods and Hollnagel 2006).

In dynamic control situations it is assumed that a so-called *controller* aims to gain and maintain control of a *process*, within a certain *environment* or context. The process is a series of changes of an object, which can be a situation, system or other phenomena. The controller has to monitor and assess the state and changes in the process to be controlled, in order to make sense of the process and form an appropriate understanding (also called model or construct) of the process (and the environment). Relying on this understanding, the controller is to determine and undertake a series of interdependent actions in order to gain and maintain control of the process, based on feedback (response) and feed-forward (prediction, anticipation). The process may change in and of itself (autonomously), due to disturbances and influences of the environment, and due to the actions of the controller. These phenomena constitute a control loop or cycle (without a fixed start or end point), which is called dynamic because of the importance of interdependent change over time in process and environment, controller understanding of these changes, and controller actions and their effects. Moreover, as the dynamic process control involves regulation of both the processes to be controlled and the controller itself, the controller has to be adaptive and have self-regulative behaviour (see Figure 6.1).

In the context of emergency and disaster response operations, a controller can be represented by a single person using technological artefacts, for instance an incident commander using different communication devices, as well as by a socio-technical system of varying complexity, for example joint command staff with personnel from a number of organizations using diverse decision-support and communication systems, or a network of command posts from which the coordination of response efforts takes place via advanced interconnected information and communication technologies.

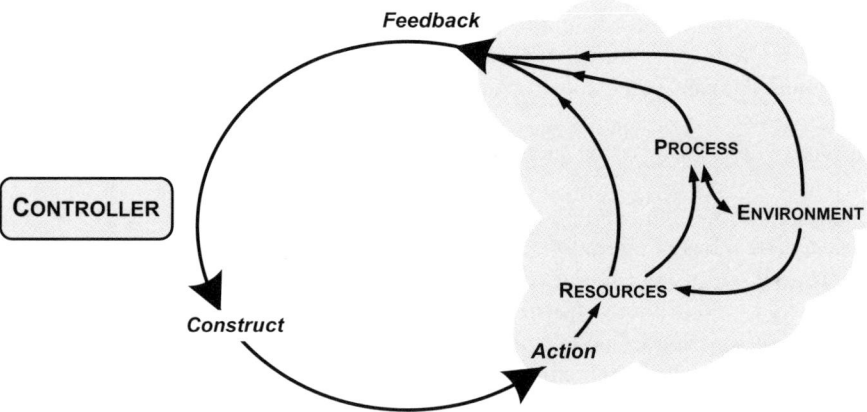

Figure 6.1   The controller acts through its resources on a process in a dynamic control loop

A similar dynamic control viewpoint has been used for describing command and control work both in emergency and disaster response as well as in the military domain (for example, Worm et al. 1998; Bakken and Gilljam 2002; Johansson and Hollnagel 2007; Svensson 2010).

Controllers are part of larger control systems
Controllers are a part of larger control systems that influence what and how specific response operations are managed and related command and control work performed.

One important characteristic of controllers managing specific response operations is that they do not act in isolation but form part of larger systems, called command and control systems. These are, in principle, permanent distributed supervisory control systems which utilize coordination of resources, controlled by the systems themselves (Shattuck and Woods 2000). Command and control systems are designed and created to support the coordination of the wide range of activities and the high number of different organizations involved in emergency and disaster response.

Control systems such as the command and control systems discussed here are characterized by highly complex and dynamic interactions and medium to low coupling between their parts (Perrow 1984). They consist of people (such as commanding officers, experts and operators), the technological artefacts they use (such as communication systems and decision-support systems) and managerial structures in which the people and technical artefacts are embedded. Command and control systems in emergency and disaster response contain various types of operational resources from diverse kinds of organizations, which have their own goals and varying operational procedures (Wybo and Lonka 2002; Schraagen and Van de Ven 2011). Moreover, individual organizations involved in emergency and disaster response may have their own command and control systems to coordinate their own operational resources. Emergency and disaster response is therefore characterized by the presence of multiple command and control systems that have different levels of interdependence (see, for example, Johansson 2010; Cedergårdh and Winnberg 2011); see Figure 6.2. For instance, fire and rescue services and police have their own command and control systems, while they may be part of other command and control systems that are generic for all types of joint operations or specific for certain risks or hazards (such as nuclear emergencies), areas (such as a particular region) or functions (such as search and rescue).

The different command and control systems are the organizational resource base from which controllers of specific response operations are established. Restrictions, limitations, regulations and other aspects related to specific command and control systems, such as allocation of authority and responsibilities, therefore set different constraints on controllers during response operations. Constraints, consequently, shape what activities are executed by controllers, and how. Not only may controllers' range of possible actions be limited; new opportunities may also be provided so that certain, initially unforeseen, actions take place (Hollnagel and Woods 2005).

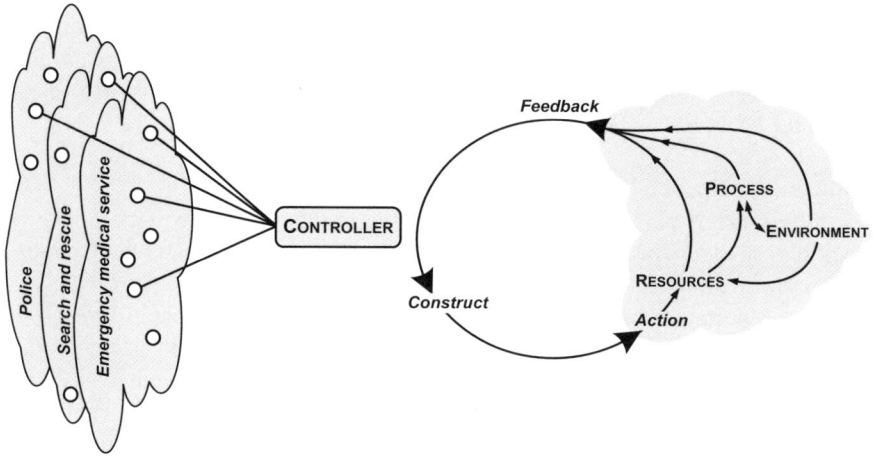

**Figure 6.2　Command and control systems contain various types of
operational resources from diverse kinds of organizations,
from which controllers are formed**

Thus, command and control work in response operations can also be seen as the
enduring management of internal and external constraints, in order to achieve
external goals defined by the multiple command and control systems, as well
as internal goals defined by the controllers. Controllers' ability to manage these
constraints and coordinate their actions accordingly determines if the controllers
are able to accomplish their tasks and, in that case, with what outcome (Persson
et al. 2000; Woltjer 2009).

Controllers are temporary, heterogeneous and task-specific
Controllers managing emergency and disaster response operations are temporary,
heterogeneous and task-specific. The viewpoint on emergency and disaster
response operations as dynamic control situations managed by a socio-technical
system means that controllers are transient. Controllers manage the progress of
ongoing emergency and disaster response operations. As the duration of any
response operation is time limited, the controllers exist on temporary bases as
well. The controllers of specific response operations are formed within minutes or
hours after the occurrence of emergencies and disasters, that is on a reactive basis
(Cedergårdh and Winnberg 2010; Schraagen and Van de Ven 2011).

The fact that controllers of response operations exist on a temporary basis
has an impact on the characteristics of the controllers in terms of the initial
conditions, as well as on the context and constraints under which the controllers
act. Controllers are organized out of the nearest available command and control
resources (personnel, technology and facilities) of the organizations involved in
the response operations and their command and control systems (as illustrated

in Figure 6.2). This means that controllers are thus configured during the initial stages of response operations, while they are already carrying out actual command and control work and manage ongoing response efforts (Svensson et al. 2009; Trnka and Johansson 2011).

Response operations are situation-driven operations where the number and type of organizations involved, the number of deployed personnel, likewise the tasks and functions performed by these organizations and personnel, as well as the interactions and relations among them, are all based on the prevailing situation and actual needs which are to be addressed. At the same time, controllers in emergency and disaster response operations are dimensioned and have command and control capacity primarily based on the same grounds. It should therefore be expected that controllers differ from response operation to response operation regarding, for example, the number of commanding personnel involved, their expertise and skills, as well as the artefacts used and, not least, controllers' internal configuration and communication (Bigley and Roberts 2001; Svensson et al. 2009; Cedergårdh and Winnberg 2010).

Controllers Need to be Adaptive in Multiple Dimensions

The third key viewpoint is centred on the dynamic nature of response operations that requires controllers to be adaptive in multiple dimensions. It is derived from the first two presented key viewpoints and the following characteristics of response operations and controllers. First, response operations, likewise the controllers managing these operations, can be unique in their setup from event to event. Second, response operations continuously change as a result of the development in the area of operations, implemented countermeasures and deployed operational resources. Thus, controllers may look different as response operations progress in terms of their size and structure, as well as in their internal coordination and the way response efforts are managed within the same response operation. Controllers must therefore be flexible and continuously adapt to these changes, as well as to shifting demands during entire response operations. In other words, controllers in emergency and disaster response operations need to be adaptive in multiple dimensions in order to accomplish their goals (see Figure 6.3). The three main dimensions of adaptation are: (a) resource-driven adaptation, (b) control-driven adaptation and (c) adaptation to unexpected disturbances and changes.

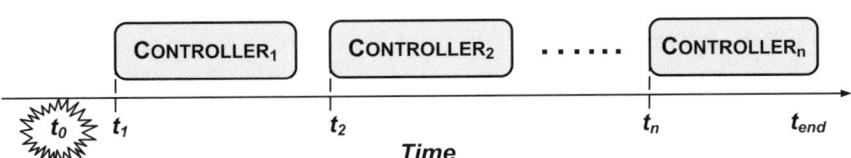

Figure 6.3 **Controllers must be flexible and continuously adapt to changes. Controllers change at different points in time, between t_0, the time of the initiating event, and t_{end}, where response operations end**

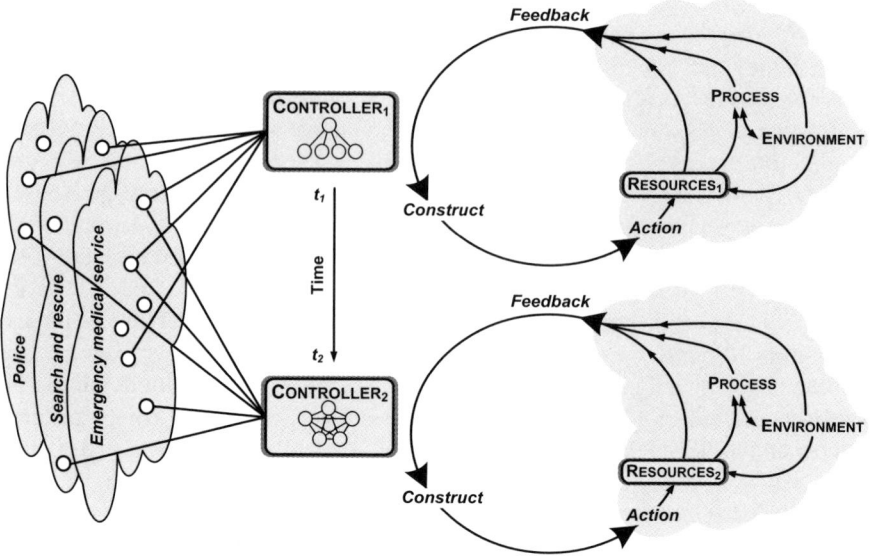

Figure 6.4   Resource-driven adaptation, where operational resources change, along with communication patterns and authority within controllers, and relations between controllers and command and control systems

Resource-driven adaptation

The nature of response operations may alter as a result of the response efforts conducted and countermeasures implemented. Consequently, the goals of controllers managing response operations may change several times during a single response operation. This means that the type and number of deployed operational resources may be continuously changing too (see, for instance, Landgren and Nulden 2007; Uhr et al. 2008; Trnka and Johansson 2011).

Controllers need to manage this complexity of emergency and disaster response operations and have a capacity to self-regulate and adapt (Fredholm 1991; Brehmer and Svenmarck 1995). They must be able to continuously adapt to these changes in terms of their size and structure to reflect these changing goals and to match the variety of the resources during the entire response operations. This corresponds to the cybernetic law of requisite variety. According to the law of requisite variety (Ashby 1956), control systems – in our case represented by controllers – should have a variety (range of actions available for process control) that at least matches the variety of the process to be controlled in the environment.

The continuous adaptation includes, for instance, the number of personnel involved, their expertise and skills, the artefacts they use and the international configuration of controllers. These changes are also equated with the shifting nature and number of relations and interactions within controllers, as well as between controllers and command and control systems, of which controllers are part. The changes may include adaptations to communication patterns and reallocation of authority (see, for example, Baber et al. 2004; Uhr et al. 2008; Cedergårdh and Winnberg 2010); see Figure 6.4.

Control-driven adaptation

Controllers managing emergency and disaster response operations often need to implement multiple countermeasures to achieve their goals. This, in combination with shifting goals, changing availability of operational resources and continuous changes in the area of operations, requires that controllers may need to be adaptive in the way they regulate the dynamic control processes to effectively manage the ongoing response operations to obtain the best possible outcome within the persisting time and resource constraints. This means they may need to utilize diverse organizational and temporal configurations of their command and control work. The organizational configurations of command and control work refer to what command and control strategies are used to effectively deploy operational resources. It also refers to the way in which command and control work is arranged to effectively coordinate countermeasures and actions put in place, as well as to how command and control work is organized in order to maintain control of deployed resources and the activities taking place. The temporary configurations refer to when and in what way controllers alter between different command and control strategies and arrangements (Fredholm 1991; Brehmer and Svenmarck 1995; Bigley and Roberts 2001; Svensson et al. 2009); see Figure 6.5.

Command and control strategies relate to how and in what way operational resources are led and coordinated, as well as how feedback on actions and countermeasures is collected. In general, three main command and control strategies can be found in response operations. These three strategies are: order-specific, task-oriented and autonomous strategy (based on Fredholm 1991; Alberts and Hayes 1995; Keithly and Ferris 1999; Lagerlöf and Pallin 1999; Alberts et al. 2001; Kaiser et al. 2004).

Order-specific command and control strategy is sometimes described as 'leading by order' as it is based on detailed and specific instructions and orders from controllers to operational resources on 'what should be done, how and when'. Order-specific command and control also requires detailed and frequent feedback on the activities taking place in the area of operations. This type of command and control strategy is recognized as coordination and communication intensive. It is often utilized, for example, in command and control of airborne operations or in situations where specific orders and instructions may be needed due to safety risks.

Task-oriented command and control strategy is characterized by general instructions that are given by controllers to operational resources on 'what should be done or achieved'. This type of strategy can be described as 'leading by task', in contrast to the order-specific command and control strategy. The instructions to operational resources take the form of directives, which include intentions, goals,

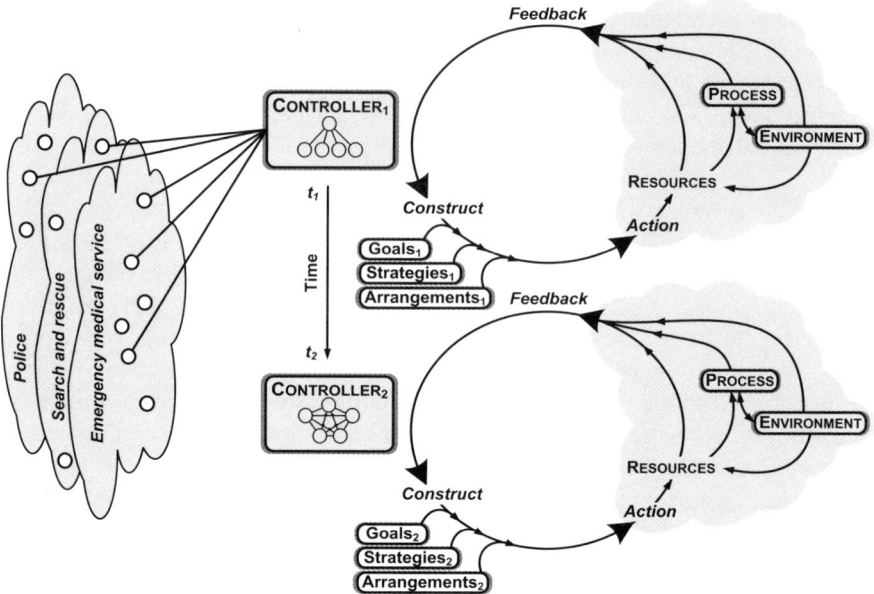

Figure 6.5   Control-driven adaptation, where controllers adapt the way they regulate the dynamic control processes by changing their communication patterns and authority allocation, goals, command and control strategies and command and control arrangements

deadlines and some guidance toward identified objectives and potential problems. The task-oriented strategy requires that operational resources are capable of taking the initiative, and choosing appropriate actions and countermeasures. This type of strategy is commonly used, for instance, by the Swedish fire and rescue services (Svensson et al. 2009).

Autonomous command and control strategy means that controllers are only concerned with general objectives such as 'save lives'. Operational resources use self-synchronization principles to choose and implement actions and countermeasures. Controllers only oversee the ongoing activities. This type of strategy utilizes high flexibility and adaptability, and is used, for instance, by the voluntary emergency medical service 'Hatzolah' in the initial stages of response operations (Kaiser et al. 2004; Piombino 2011).

The different command and control strategies require various competences, skills and capacities. The choice of a command and control strategy depends on a given situation, but also on the skills, competence and experience of the command and control personnel involved, as well as on the training, skills and capacities of the deployed operational resources. There are also qualitative and quantitative differences between these three command and control strategies (see Table 6.1), which do not make the strategies equally applicable to all situations. The task-oriented and autonomous command and control strategies may not be suitable for all circumstances, for instance where the activities taking place are interrelated or restrained by the same type of constraints, or where the deployed operational resources do not have local knowledge or sufficient skills for the specific tasks they are supposed to execute. On the other hand, the order-specific command and control strategy that allows deployment of less-skilled or experienced operational resources has, at the same time, higher coordination and communication demands compared to the task-oriented and autonomous command and control strategies (see, for instance, Johansson 2000; Cedergårdh and Winnberg 2010).

Table 6.1   A comparison of the three different command and control strategies with respect to feedback, command and resource attributes

	Feedback attributes		Command attributes		Resource attributes	
	Level of detail	Frequency	Level of detail	Frequency	Competence / skills	Creativity / initiative
Order-specific	*Low*	*Low*	*Low*	*Low*	*Very high*	*Very high*
Task-oriented	*Moderate*	*Moderate*	*Moderate / high*	*Moderate / high*	*Moderate / high*	*Moderate / high*
Autonomous	*High*	*Very high*	*Moderate*	*High*	*Moderate / low*	*Moderate / low*

Source: Based on Alberts and Hayes (1995); Alberts et al. (2001).

While command and control strategies relate to how and in what way operational resources are led and coordinated, command and control arrangements concern how command and control is organized with respect to operational resources and the area of operations in order to achieve *unity of direction* in command and control work. In principle, there are three basic approaches: geography-, function- and domain-based arrangements (based on Fredholm 1991; Johansson 2000; Brunacini 2002; Walsh et al. 2005; Cedergårdh and Winnberg 2010).

  Geography-based arrangements mean that activities in the area of operations are disposed according to the geography. In other words, operational resources are allocated in geographical sectors where each sector contains commonly all resources that are necessary to accomplish goals related to specific sectors. In *function-based arrangements* operational resources are allocated to support specific activities such as pumping, search and rescue or evacuations, throughout the entire area of operations. *Domain-based arrangements* organize resources based on organizations' domain of competence, for example, police forces, emergency medical services and fire and rescue services, over the entire area of operations.

The different types of command and control arrangements are often combined in various ways. For instance, the domain-based arrangements, for example fire and rescue, emergency medical services, police, and so forth, can be used to structure the overall coordination of all operational resources in the area of operations. The function-based arrangements can then be used at the same time within each domain, for instance, police allocating their resources to surveillance, patrolling and victim identification. Similar to the command and control strategies, the different command and control arrangements are different with respect to coordination and communication requirements and are not equally applicable to all situations. For instance, the function-based arrangements are suitable for situations where there are uneven tasks, coordination and communication load on the different activities being conducted. On the other hand, the geography-based arrangements can be used in situations where a large number of operational resources in different sectors perform activities that are not related to or not dependent on activities in the other sectors.

In order to effectively deploy operational resources and coordinate response efforts, controllers may adapt organizational and temporal configurations of their command and control work by implementing different command and control strategies and arrangements. Controllers may use and switch between the different strategies and arrangements, and that way influence the number and range of activities and resources they are capable to coordinate. Depending on prevailing circumstances controllers may choose to use temporally specific command and control strategies and arrangements, for instance in order to reduce communication and work load on dedicated command and control functions, or to allow deployment of certain operational resources. Controllers may employ specific command and control strategies and arrangements to establish safety for personnel in the area of operations, or to cope with disturbances in communication, as another example. Such adaptations may be pre-planned and based on informal doctrines and procedures, such as the so-called incident command system, or emerge on an ad hoc basis (see, for example, Baber et al. 2004; Militello et al. 2007; Svensson et al. 2009; Alberts et al. 2010).

Adaptation to unexpected disturbances and changes
As suggested in the first two dimensions of adaptation, controllers in emergency and disaster response operations need to be prepared for a great deal of adaptation and flexibility as part of their competence and ordinary working methods. However, as it is practically impossible to foresee all possible thinkable and unthinkable scenarios and situations, controllers must be able to go beyond established forms of prepared-for adaptation and be able to adapt to unexpected disturbances and changes as well. This means they must be resilient and able to improvise.

To be resilient means that controllers are able to handle unforeseen disturbances and variations. In other words, controllers have to be able to anticipate and mitigate potential scenarios and situations that may lead to disruptions of response efforts, as well as to identify and cope with disruptions already taking place. Controllers also have to be able to recover from disruptions that have not been anticipated or properly coped with (see, for instance, Westrum 2006; Hollnagel 2009).

In order to achieve resilient response, controllers may employ dynamic management of response operations, that is using shifting responsibilities and reallocation of authority in order to better respond to changing circumstances and demands (see Figures 6.4 and 6.5). Controllers may, therefore, to a certain extent, accept inefficient management of response efforts in the short term in order to maintain flexibility and be able to meet variations that may occur during response operations and ensure long-term effectiveness (see, for example, Nylén 1996; Militello et al. 2007; Branlat et al. 2009; Woods and Branlat 2010).

As a result of the novelty of situations faced by controllers, some form of improvisation is usually necessary (Mendonça and Wallace 2004). Improvisation refers to controllers' management of situations where (a) no plan or procedure applies under prevailing circumstances, or (b) an existing plan or procedure cannot be executed. The actual level of improvisation may range from modest adjustments of applicable procedures to complete abandonment of all (pre-)existing plans and procedures (see, for example, Moorman and Miner 1998). This may imply selecting and executing one or more alternative courses of action, developing and deploying one or several new procedures, or taking on new roles (Mendonça and Wallace 2007). Improvisation may also imply adjustments of command and control work in terms of internal communication and coordination, task allocation or overall management approach (Mendonça and Fiedrich 2006; Mendonça and Wallace 2007; Rankin et al. 2013). Thus, beyond established forms of prepared-for adaptations, controllers may employ a varying degree of improvisation, enabling controllers to adapt on a sliding scale of extent of adaptation; see Figure 6.6.

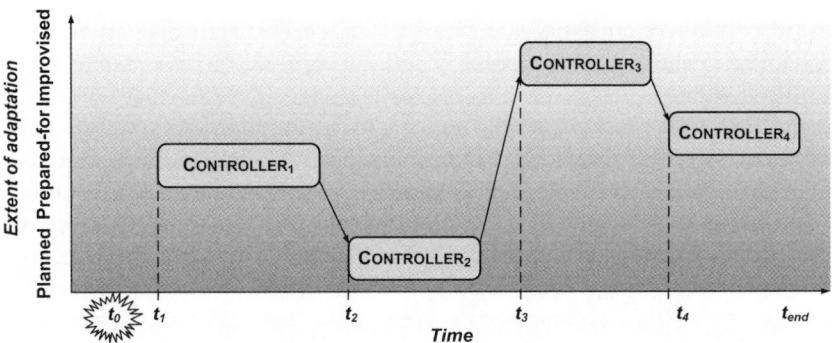

Figure 6.6   **Controllers adapt over time to a varying extent, ranging from planned, to prepared-for, to improvised work forms**

Discussion and Concluding Remarks

This section discusses the described main characteristics of emergency and disaster response operations and related command and control work. It also discusses differences and commonalities between command and control in emergency and disaster response and military operations, as well as their implications for joint operations.

We have presented three key viewpoints on which basis we discuss emergency and disaster response operations and related command and control work. By using these key viewpoints we have identified the following main characteristics of emergency and disaster response operations.

First, emergency and disaster response operations are of a need-based character. They are governed by actual needs in particular response operations, which influence which organizations will be involved, to what extent, as well as how the operations will be organized. They may, therefore, to a large extent be unique in their setup from emergency to emergency or disaster to disaster.

Second, command and control structures (described in this chapter as controllers) in charge of particular response operations are transient entities. They are organized shortly after an emergency or disaster has taken place (within minutes or hours) out of the nearest available command and control resources of the involved organizations and their command and control systems. They are established 'on the run' during the initial stages of response operations with a reactive and bottom-up approach. Their command and control work is influenced by the presence of multiple command and control systems that are heterogeneous and have different levels of interdependence. They are disbanded as the response operations are concluded. Controllers managing particular operations thus exist only for short periods of time (hours to days; in extreme cases, weeks). As a result, which command and control resources will be involved, to what extent, for how long, as well as how they will be organized, may not be fully determined in advance.

Third, controllers managing emergency and disaster response operations are not stable entities. Instead they continuously adjust to shifting demands and changing circumstances throughout the entire response operations. This adaptation takes place in multiple dimensions. It may include, for instance, changes in the number of command and control personnel involved and the allocation of tasks. It may be equated with a shifting of communication patterns and reallocation of authority. The adaptation may also concern use of diverse organizational and temporal configurations of command and control work over time. Unplanned adjustments in courses of actions or improvised deployments of procedures are another example.

Based on these main characteristics we argue that military operations and emergency and disaster response operations are different in many aspects. For instance, controllers in charge of military operations are commonly established in advance, over a period of weeks or months. They are dimensioned largely based on planning using a top-down approach. They often have explicitly specified structures, allocation of authority, communication channels and so on. Further, they are established from the command and control resources of a single organization and its single command and control system, or alternatively of a limited number of organizations and a limited number of homogeneous command and control systems. During military operations controllers may adjust to shifting demands and changing circumstances too; however, the degree and frequency of these adjustments is different compared to emergency and disaster response operations.

If military organizations take part in emergency and disaster response operations, or conduct joint operations with emergency and disaster response organizations, they need to be aware of the qualitative and quantitative differences in the way emergency and disaster response operations are organized and managed. They need to be prepared for the emergency and disaster response organizations to continuously adjust their command and control work in multiple dimensions. Therefore, military organizations may need to accept that the level of transparency and predictability of response operations and command and control work may not be at the level they are used to from military operations. Moreover, they may be forced to adjust in similar ways to the emergency response organizations and their command and control structures in order to conduct joint operations.

References

Alberts, D.S., Garstka, J.J., Hayes, R.E. and Signori, D.A. (2001). *Understanding Information Age Warfare*. Washington DC: The Command and Control Research Program.

Alberts, D.S. and Hayes, R.E. (1995). *Command Arrangements for Peace Operations*. Washington DC: The Command and Control Research Program.

Alberts, D.S., Huber, R.K. and Moffat, J. (2010). *NATO NEC C2 Maturity Model*. Washington DC: The Command and Control Research Program.

Ashby, W.R. (1956). *An Introduction to Cybernetics*. London: Chapman & Hall.

Baber, C., Houghton, R.J., McMaster, R., Salmon, P., Stanton, N.A., Stewart, R.J. and Walker, G.H. (2004). *Field Studies in the Emergency Services*. HFIDTC/WP1.1.1/1-1. Yeovil: Human Factors Integration Defence Technology Centre.

Bakken, B.T. and Gilljam, M. (2002). Dynamic intuition in military command and control: Why it is important, and how it should be developed. *Cognition, Technology & Work*, 5(3), 197–205.

Bigley, G.A. and Roberts, K.H. (2001). The incident command system: High-reliability organizing for complex and volatile task environments. *Academy of Management Journal*, 44(6), 1281–99.

Branlat, M., Fern, L., Voshell, M. and Trent, S. (2009). Understanding coordination challenges in urban firefighting: A study of critical incident reports. *Proceedings of the Human Factors and Ergonomics Society Annual Meeting*, 53(4), 284–8.

Brehmer, B. (1992). Dynamic decision making: Human control of complex systems. *Acta Psychologica*, 81(3), 211–41.

Brehmer, B. and Allard, R. (1991). Real-time dynamic decision making: The effects of task complexity and feedback delays. In J. Rasmussen, B. Brehmer and J. Leplat (eds), *Distributed Decision Making: Cognitive Models for Cooperative Work*. Chichester: John Wiley & Sons, 319–34.

Brehmer, B. and Svenmarck, P. (1995). Distributed decision making in dynamic environments: Time scales and architectures of decision making. In J.-P. Caverni, M. Bar-Hillel, F.H. Barron and H. Jungermann (eds), *Contributions to Decision Making – I*. Amsterdam: Elsevier Science, 155–74.

Brunacini, A.V. (2002). *Fire Command: The Essential of Local IMS*, 2nd ed. Quincy, MA: U.S. National Fire Protection Association.

Cedergårdh, E. and Winnberg, T. (2010). Structuring a command organization. In L. Fredholm and A.-L. Göransson (eds), *Emergency Response Management in Today's Complex Society*. Karlstad: Swedish Civil Contingencies Agency, 197–248.

Cedergårdh, E. and Winnberg, T. (2011). Proaktiv samverkan vid olyckor (In Swedish). In N.-O. Nilsson, J. Gert, T. Johansson, L.-G. Emanuelsson, K. Pedersen, S. Lind and G. Berg (eds), *Samverkan – för säkerhets skull!*. Karlstad: Swedish Civil Contingencies Agency, 81–104.

Comfort, L.K., Sungu, Y., Johnson, D. and Dunn, M. (2001). Complex systems in crisis: Anticipation and resilience in dynamic environments. *Journal of Contingencies and Crisis Management*, 8(4), 208–17.

Davidson, L.W., Hayes, M.D. and Landon, J.J. (1996). *Humanitarian and Peace Operations: NGO and the Military in the Interagency Process*. Washington DC: The Command and Control Research Program.

Drabek, T.E. and McEntire, D.A. (2003). Emergent phenomena and the sociology of a disaster. *Disaster Prevention and Management*, 12(2), 97–112.

Fredholm, L. (1991). *The Development of Rescue Tactics: Analysis and Proposed Methods*. FOA Report C 500895.3. Sundbyberg, Sweden: National Defence Research Establishment.

Fredholm, L. (2010). Dealing with all types of emergency from everyday accidents up to disasters. In L. Fredholm and A.–L. Göransson (eds), *Emergency Response Management in Today's Complex Society*. Karlstad: Swedish Civil Contingencies Agency, 13–30.

Hicks, E.K. and Pappas, G. (2006). Coordinating disaster relief after the South Asia earthquake. *Society*, 43(5), 42–50.

Hollnagel, E. (1998). Context, cognition, and control. In Y. Waern (ed.), *Co-operation in Process Management: Cognition and Information Technology*. London: Taylor & Francis, 27–51.

Hollnagel, E. (2009). The four cornerstones of resilience engineering. In E. Hollnagel and S. Dekker (eds), *Resilience Engineering Perspectives, Vol. 2 – Preparation and Restoration*. Farnham: Ashgate, 117–33.

Hollnagel, E. and Woods, D.D. (2005). *Joint Cognitive Systems: Foundations of Cognitive Systems Engineering*. Boca Raton, FL: CRC Press/Taylor & Francis.

Johansson, P. (2000). *Effektiv insatsledning – några teoretiska grunder för ledning av polis – och räddningsinsatser* (In Swedish). Karlstad: Swedish Rescue Services Agency.

Johansson, P. (2010). Legal grounds for emergency response operations. In L. Fredholm and A.-L. Göransson (eds), *Emergency Response Management in Today's Complex Society*. Karlstad: Swedish Civil Contingencies Agency, 151–84.

Johansson, B. and Hollnagel, E. (2007). Pre-requisites for large scale coordination. *Cognition, Technology & Work*, 9(1), 5–13.

Kaiser, M., Larsson, P. and Hörnsten-Friberg, L. (2004). *Krishantering med en vidgad syn på nätverksorganisering* (In Swedish). FOI-R-1248-SE. Stockholm: Swedish Defence Research Agency.

Keithly, D.M. and Ferris, S.P. (1999). Auftragstaktik, or directive control, in joint and combined operations. *Parameters*, 29(3), 118–33.

Kendra, J.M. and Wachtendorf, T. (2006). *Improvisation, Creativity, and the Art of Emergency Management*. DRC Preliminary Paper #357. Newark, DE: University of Delaware.

Lagerlöf, J. and Pallin, K. (1999). Doctrine and command in the Swedish armed forces. In *Proceedings of the CCRTS Command and Control Research and Technology Symposium*. Newport, RI.

Landgren, J. and Nulden, U. (2007). A study of emergency response work: Patterns of mobile phone interaction. In M.B. Rosson and D. Gilmore (eds), *Proceedings of the SIGCHI Conference on Human Factors in Computing Systems*. New York: ACM Press, 1323–32.

McEntire, D.A. (1999). Issues in disaster relief: Progress, perceptual problems and prospective solutions. *Disaster Prevention and Management*, 8(5), 351–61.

Mendonça, D. and Fiedrich, F. (2006). Training for improvisation in emergency management: Opportunities and limits for information technology. *International Journal of Emergency Management*, 3(4), 348–63.

Mendonça, D. and Wallace, W.A. (2004). Studying organizationally situated improvisation in response to extreme events. *International Journal of Mass Emergencies and Disasters*, 22(2), 5–29.

Mendonça, D. and Wallace, W.A. (2007). A cognitive model of improvisation in emergency management. *IEEE Transactions on Systems, Man and Cybernetics, Part A*, 37(4), 547–61.

Militello, L.G., Patterson, E.S., Bowman, L. and Wears, R. (2007). Information flow during crisis management: Challenges to coordination in the emergency operations center. *Cognition, Technology & Work*, 9(1), 25–31.

Moorman, C. and Miner, A.S. (1998). Organizational improvisation and organizational memory. *The Academy of Management Review*, 23(4), 698–723.

Neisser, U. (1976). *Cognition and Reality: Principles and Implications of Cognitive Psychology*. San Francisco, CA: W.H. Freeman and Company.

Nylén, L. (1996). The role of the police in the total management of disaster. *Disaster Prevention and Management*, 5(5), 23–30.

Perrow, C. (1984). *Normal Accidents: Living with High-risk Technologies*. New York: Basic Books.

Persson, P.-A., Nyce, J.M. and Eriksson, H. (2000). Command and control: A biased combination? In C. McCann and R. Pigeau (eds), *The Human in Command: Exploring the Modern Military Experience*. New York: Kluwer Academic/Plenum Publishers, 201–16.

Piombino, A.E. (2011). Hatzalah: 'Extreme' faith-based emergency responders. *IAEM Bulletin*, 28(10), 36–7.

Quarantelli, E.L. (1993). *Technological and Natural Disasters and Ecological Problems: Similarities and Differences in Planning for and Managing Them*. DRC Prelimary Paper #192. Newark, DE: University of Delaware.

Quarantelli, E.L. (2000). *Emergencies, Disaster and Catastrophes are Different Phenomena*. DRC Preliminary Paper #304. Newark, DE: University of Delaware.

Quarantelli, E.L. (2003). *A Half Century of Social Science Disaster Research: Selected Major Findings and Their Applicability*. DRC Preliminary Paper #336. Newark, DE: University of Delaware.

Rankin, A., Dahlbäck, N. and Lundberg, J. (2013). A case study of factors influencing role improvisation in crisis response teams. *Cognition, Technology & Work*, 15(1), 79–93.

Schraagen, J.M. and Van de Ven, J. (2011). Human factors aspects of ICT for crisis management. *Cognition, Technology & Work*, 13(3), 175–87.

Shattuck, L. and Woods, D.D. (2000). Communication of intent in military command and control systems. In C. McCann and R. Pigeau (eds), *The Human in Command: Exploring the Modern Military Experience*. New York: Kluwer Academic/Plenum Publishers, 279–92.

Suparamaniam, N. and Dekker, S. (2003). Paradoxes of power: The separation of knowledge and authority in international disaster relief work. *Disaster Prevention and Management*, 12(4), 312–18.

Svensson, S. (2010). The theory of fundamental tactics. In L. Fredholm and A.-L. Göransson (eds), *Emergency Response Management in Today's Complex Society*. Karlstad: Swedish Civil Contingencies Agency, 185–96.

Svensson, S., Cedergårdh, E., Mårtensson O. and Winnberg, T. (2009). *Tactics, Command, Leadership*. Karlstad: Swedish Civil Contingencies Agency.

Trnka, J. and Johansson, B. (2011). Resilient emergency response: Supporting flexibility and improvisation in collaborative command and control. In M.E. Jennex (ed.), *Crisis Response and Management and Emerging Information Systems: Critical Applications*. Hershey, PA: IGI Global, 112–38.

Uhr, C., Johansson, H. and Fredholm, L. (2008). Analysing emergency response systems. *Journal of Contingencies and Crisis Management*, 16(2), 80–90.

Walsh, D.W., Christen, H.T. Jr., Miller, G.T., Callsen, C.E. Jr., Cilluffo, F.J. and Maniscalo, P.M. (2005). *National Incident Management System: Principles and Practice*. Sudbury, MA: Jones and Barlett Publishers.

Westtrum, R. (2006). A typology of resilience situations. In E. Hollnagel, D.D. Woods and N. Levenson (eds), *Resilience Engineering: Concepts and Precepts*. Aldershot: Ashgate, 55–65.

Wiener, N. (1948). *Cybernetics or Control and Communication in the Animal and the Machine*. Cambridge, MA: MIT Press.

Woltjer, R. (2009). *Functional Modeling of Constraint Management in Aviation Safety and Command and Control*. Dissertation No. 1249, Linköping Studies in Science and Technology. Linköping, Sweden: Linköpings universitet.

Woods, D.D. and Branlat, M. (2010). Hollnagel's test: Being 'in control' of highly interdependent multi-layered networked systems. *Cognition, Technology & Work*, 12(2), 95–101.

Woods, D.D. and Hollnagel, E. (2006). *Joint Cognitive Systems: Patterns in Cognitive Systems Engineering*. Boca Raton, FL: CRC Press/Taylor & Francis.

Worm, A., Jenvald, J. and Morin, M. (1998). Mission efficiency analysis: Evaluating and improving tactical mission performance in high-risk, time-critical operations. *Safety Science*, 30(1–2), 79–98.

Wybo, J.-L. and Lonka, H. (2002). Emergency management and information society: How to improve synergy? *International Journal of Emergency Management*, 1(2), 183–90.

Chapter 7

Empirical Studies of Command and Control Centres at the Swedish Air Force

E. Svensson, C. Rencrantz, J. Marklund and P. Berggren

Introduction

The problem of measuring and assessing complex command and control environments to better understand them, or to get performance measures for training and validation of novel systems and methods, is well known. It is easily assumed that it would be easier to measure these matters as modern systems have better capabilities for recording what happens. Yet, the inherent complexity and dynamics of command and control situations *is* very challenging. This experience is repeated whenever armed forces all over the world, as well as large-scale crisis management actors, need feedback on how they are doing, and feed-forward on how they will do. It is often the case that technical command and control systems cannot provide them with answers.

As discussed in Chapter 4, techniques of measurement reflect the status at a certain time (or for a period of time), or they can reflect dynamic changes or processes over time. The two types of technique complement each other and reflect different aspects of, for example, command and control processes, although capturing the dynamic changes of a command and control situation may be an endeavour more challenging than that for stable or slow-change situations. Different situational challenges call for different measuring techniques; dynamic environments, indeed, demand dynamic measures. Even at a low level of complexity it may be difficult to reach solid and reliable assessments of command and control processes (Essens et al. 2005).

A command and control environment is a dynamic and complex setting with interacting systems and teams of operators. The resemblance to natural decision-making, as described in the literature (Klein et al. 1993; Klein 1999), is obvious (changing goals, high stakes, time stress, constraints and dynamic settings). To know when such teams and systems perform well is crucial for system verification, validation and the training of command and control teams. Repeated measurement is also of imperative importance for predicting changes in complex and dynamic events. Using predictions of changes as regards, for example, mental workload, performance, adaptability of teams, sub-teams and positions can be identified and/ or carried out.

It is important to consider the dynamics of technical and human aspects of command and control. No matter how complex, interactions between technical and human systems over time generate essential information and, to some extent, forecast operators' workload and performance.

If it was possible, it would be convenient to assess operational studies in the same way as classical experiments, that is, using a limited number of specified variables allowing controlled comparisons. It is not possible to approach and study many dynamic situations with classical experimental design, however, due to their complexity. If too much control is imposed, the realism and dynamics are lost. Therefore, from a practical (applied) point of view, it is desirable to assess experts in their natural, dynamic environments, during training sessions, operational field exercises or other similar circumstances. In such cases, it is virtually impossible to interfere with or actively manipulate actions, so methods have to be adjusted. Fortunately, second-generation multivariate statistics make it possible to draw scientifically valid conclusions from studies of situations characterized by high realism and complexity.

Naturalistic observation is a practical analytical solution for the assessment of dynamic variables. Subject matter experts (or instructors) are often obliged to evaluate participants' performance in complex training sessions. A recurring problem, however, is that it is difficult to involve a sufficient number of instructors due to economical and practical restrictions. One way of handling this is to let operators themselves assess matters such as mental workload, situational awareness and performance as, after all, workload and situational awareness are, partially, internal mental processes and, thereby, not easily available, nor directly observable. This type of analytical management is appropriate in regard to earlier research as several studies show that there are manifest correlations between operators' own assessments of, for example, performance on the one hand and objective or instructors' measures of performance on the other hand (Angelborg-Thanderz 1997; Smith-Jentsch et al. 1998; Berggren 2000, 2005; Silverman 2001).

In the following, we present two examples of assessments of dynamic performance (hence different aspects thereof) in operational command and control situations. The first study was carried out at the command and control centre of the Swedish Air Force (StriC in Uppsala; see, for example, Svensson et al. 2006; Paris et al. 2011). One general purpose of this study was to test and develop evaluation techniques for complex environments, to validate the techniques and to demonstrate their practicability in operational settings. Another purpose of this first study was to train Swedish operators with respect to interoperability in NATO. In both cases, these were problems that the Swedish Armed Forces needed to address. The study was conducted in an operational command and control environment where professionals with different roles, tasks and sub-goals worked as teams.

The second study took place at the Swedish Armed Forces' Control and Reporting Centre (CRC) in Skåne (see Rencrantz et al. 2007). The purpose of this study was to describe the work process of the CRC, to identify problems and to explicitly suggest improvements to the ordinary work process, all essential for the Swedish Armed Forces. The focus was on describing how central concepts such as workload, situational awareness and (aspects of) performance change over time. In both studies, data were collected so-called quasi-dynamically by means of questionnaires, in this case on personal digital assistants (PDAs). This implies that the measures were discrete even if the underlying psychological variables (such as, for example, heart rate,) by definition are continuous and dynamic (see Chapter 4).

Quasi-dynamic, or repeated measurement techniques with discrete scale formats, have been used in earlier studies (see Svensson et al. 1997b; Berggren 2000; Nählinder and Berggren 2002; Dahlström and Nählinder 2009) as well as in validation studies of Swedish Armed Forces' military aircraft systems (Svensson and Angelborg-Thanderz 2000).

Method

The first study, as described above, was conducted in a Combined Air Operations Centre (CAOC) in Uppsala, as part of a trilateral cooperation between the Netherlands, Canada and Sweden, while the second study took place at the Swedish Armed Forces' Control and Reporting Centre (CRC) in Skåne. Operators from the Swedish Armed Forces participated in both studies. In the first case, a peace support operation scenario in an operational setting (called DONFOR) constituted empirical material; in the second case, ordinary operational activities at the CRC, in Skåne, were studied.

Participants

The participants in the first study were officers from the Swedish Armed Forces operating in a CRC and a CAOC. The CRC involved one master controller (MC), one fighter allocator (CFSL), two fighter controllers (FSL), two track production officers (MRO) and one land component allocator (SAM). The CAOC consisted of one current operations officer (here referred to as CAOC) and one chief current operations officer (here referred to as CCAOC). In addition to these, one person represented the land component (a SAM allocator). Altogether nine participants (eight men, one woman) took active part in the first study. These participants were all experienced officers accomplishing tasks similar to those in their daily work. Navy, air and land components were simulated by game personnel. Representatives from the Netherlands and Canada participated in the study too, two of them as command and control instructors and two as specialists with respect to NATO standards and routines.

The participants in the second study were officers from the Swedish Armed Forces stationed at (operating) the CRC in Skåne. At any moment of the study, six positions (one master controller, four fighter controllers and one fighter allocator) were in focus. In all, four groups of six operators of the CRC participated.

Material

The first study (the Uppsala study) was conducted with regular systems and simulation equipment. This implies that every operator used his/her own platform consisting of two computer screens, keyboard and mouse. These platforms were linked so that all operators could access information from one other, as well as from the system which, in turn, was equal to that of their everyday professional work. In the second study (the Skåne study), the regular system and standard operational procedures were used by the CRC operators. The operator platforms were linked in the same way as in the first study.

As regards the questionnaire, its short and concise questions were answered on PDAs (specifically HP Pocket PC 4700 and Qtec Pocket PC 9090). In the Uppsala study, the questions aimed at capturing aspects of performance, workload, situation awareness, complexity, team coordination and sharing of information. In the Skåne study, the questionnaire also included questions concerning common understanding, tediousness, distribution of work and shift change. In the first study, participants answered items every 10 minutes. Because of the low intensity of information flow in the second study, participants answered items every 30 minutes during daytime and once an hour during night-time.

Scenario

The first study built on cooperation between different staffs, in different countries, so that a peace support operation could be executed. The scenario was based on a conflict between two fictive countries called St Donica and Noriéga.[1] The conflict is about the island Lazora, rich on oil, situated between the two countries. Officially, Lazora belongs to St Donica, but Noriéga denies Lazora's status. The military threat from Noriéga escalates, although the UN Security Council officially demands Noriéga's acknowledgement (Noriéga denies). Consequently, the UN starts a peace enforcement operation called DONFOR. This operation, lasting for four days, is led by Sweden with assisting personnel from Canada and the Netherlands. The goal of the operation is to create stability in the area, and to ensure that infringements of St Donica come to an end. At the beginning of the week, there are many non-critical incidents or routine events that the operators normally face on a daily, regular basis. During the week, however, the conflict escalates, ending in full-scale war.

---

1 Apparent similarities can be seen between this scenario and NATO's scenario: 'SKOLKAN: Scandinavia's alter ego'. *The Three Swords Magazine*, 21, 2011.

The second study answered Swedish Armed Forces' questions on operational efficiency and also formed part of the ongoing improvement process of their control and reporting centres. Accordingly, it was performed in a Swedish Armed Forces CRC during ordinary routine working conditions, meaning non-stop (24 hours) for five days.

Procedure

The first study was conducted over the course of four days. The first day was devoted to preparation and training; the remaining three days to data collection. Data were collected by means of digital questionnaires answered by the participants on PDAs every 10 minutes. This design enabled dynamic measurement in terms of time series indicating how the scenario and the situation developed, and also how it affected the participants' situational awareness, workload and performance, all in relation to time and situational requirements. All questions in the first study were extracted from exploratory studies and related to the complexity of the scenario, workload, situation awareness, performance, information sharing and team coordination.

In the second study, questions concerning common understanding, tediousness, distribution of work and shift change were added. The questions of both studies were answered on a scale format from 1 (very low/bad) to 5 (very high/good). For example: how high was your mental workload during the last time sequence?

Having presented the data and the circumstances for the recordings, we proceed with the analytical procedures. Due to the repeated measurement design, the data bases of both studies are extensive, and data reduction techniques are called for. By means of these techniques a larger number of variables are reduced to a smaller number of factors or dimensions. So-called time series require specific analyses before data reduction, and appropriate techniques for this will be used. As a second step after data reduction, we will analyse the causal relations between the factors, and for this we use techniques for empirical modelling. To reduce error variance and to give clarifying visual presentations of time series, smoothing and curve-fitting techniques will be used. By means of these statistical techniques our complex and large data bases will be transformed to simple and clarifying models and curves. It is to be observed that there is no loss of information in the transformations performed by means of these statistical techniques.

Statistical Techniques

Factor analysis (FA) is an analytical technique that makes it possible to reduce a larger number of interrelated manifest variables to a smaller number of latent variables or factors. The technique is based on the covariation of manifest measured variables. Its goal is to achieve a simplified description of data by using the smallest number of explanatory concepts needed to explain the maximum amount of common variance in a correlation matrix, that is, a table showing the intercorrelations of manifest variables (Hair et al. 1998).

Dynamic factor analysis (DFA) is a technique appropriate for multivariate time series. In contrast to classical FA, with factors showing inter-individual variance, DFA factors present intra-individual variance. Accordingly, there is an important difference between classical and dynamic factor analyses in the input matrix. In classical FA, the input matrix represents concurrent covariances, or correlations between a set of variables extracted from a sample of subjects. In DFA, on the other hand, the input matrix not only represents concurrent correlations, but also the lagged relations (or correlations) between time series variables. In contrast to classical FA, thus, DFA can be performed on time series data from one or more subject (Nesselroade and Molenaar 2004; Molenaar 2006).

Turning to structural equation modelling (SEM), the linear structural relationship and the factor structure are combined into one comprehensive model suitable for observational studies. The connections between the latent constructs (or factors) compose this structural model. More specifically, the relationships between the latent constructs and their observable indicators compose the factor or measurement model. Analysis of linear structural relationships (LISREL) is a general and flexible program for structural equation modelling analysis which generates a series of so-called goodness of fit measures for the whole model (Jöreskog and Sörbom 1993; Hair et al. 1998). A detailed description of the statistical techniques presented above is presented in Chapter 4.

Examples of psychological models developed in LISREL are given in Svensson et al. (1993, 1997a), Svensson (1997), Berggren (2000), Svensson and Wilson (2002), Nählinder et al. (2004), Castor (2009) and Nählinder (2009).

The analytical data reduction and modelling tools were applied according to the following process. First, we grouped the variables to factors; second, we developed a general and static model of the factors; third, the static model was transformed to a dynamic model.

Results

In the first study, data in terms of time series (using PDAs) were repeatedly collected from all participants, in total 48 times during the scenario. The six markers used were mental workload, scenario complexity, situational awareness, individual performance, team coordination and information sharing. By means of factor analyses of the intra-individual variance, as well as inter-individual variance, a causal model was developed

As can be seen in Figure 7.1, the markers of the workload factor are the items mental workload and scenario complexity. The markers of the individual performance factor are the items situational awareness and individual performance, whereas the markers of the team performance factor are the items team coordination and information sharing. To clarify, Figure 7.1 shows a model of the causal relations between the three factors mental workload, individual performance and team performance. Workload correlates negatively with individual performance and individual performance correlates positively with team performance. This implies that if an operator manages a high workload, this affects his/her individual performance negatively which, in turn, affects team performance negatively. The reliability (Cronbach's alpha, which is a reliability coefficient that describes how well a group of items focuses on a construct, as well as its inter-item consistency) is .83 for workload, .81 for individual performance and .85 for team performance. The goodness of fit indices of the SEM model are as follows: weighted least squares chi-square = 14.89, df = 7 and *p* = 0.04. The root mean square error of approximation (RMSEA) = 0.053, the comparative fit index (CFI) = 0.99 and the normed fit index (NFI) = .99. Taken together, the indices presented above indicate that the statistical fit of the model is high. This means that the correlations between the six different markers can be fully explained by the three different factors and their causal relationships. The CFI shows, for example, that 99 per cent of the covariance between the markers is explained by the model.

In Figure 7.1, the manifest variables are Ment. WL = mental workload, Complexity = scenario complexity, SA = situational awareness, Ind. Performance = individual performance, Team coor. = team coordination, Info. sharing = information sharing.

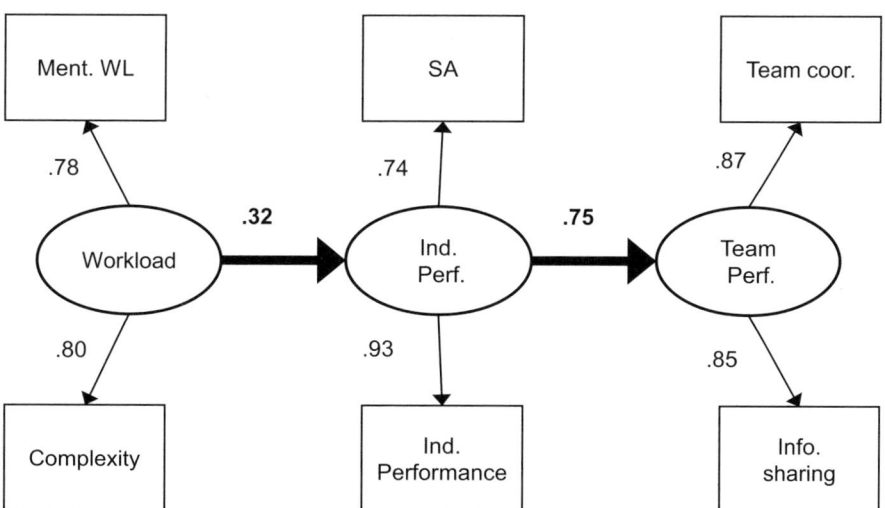

Figure 7.1   **Model of the causal relations between the factors mental workload (Workload), individual performance (Ind. Perf.) and team performance (Team Perf.)**

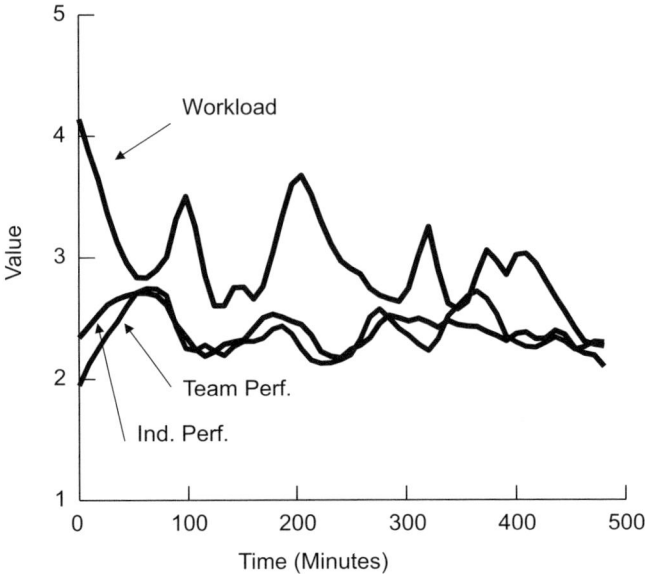

Figure 7.2   Changes in workload (Workload), individual performance (Ind. Perf.) and team performance (Team Perf.) as a function of time and situational complexity

Figure 7.2 illustrates the dynamics of the workload and performance measures as a function of time and scenario situation. In order to reduce error variance and to give a clarifying visual presentation, the curves have been smoothed by means of distant weighted least squares regression (DWLS; Wilkinson 1996). This second figure illustrates that there is an inverse relation between workload and performance measures. Performance increases when workload decreases, and vice versa. As an example, the workload increase and performance decrease during the period 160–200 minutes manifests a change from 'peace' to 'high alert'. Figure 7.2, further, shows the close relationship between the performance measures caused by the strong effect of individual performance on team performance. As much as 56 per cent of the team's performance variation can be explained by the performance of the individual. Furthermore, workload (in contrast to performance) seems to present a downward trend over the scenario development. The downward trend indicates that mental workload decreases in spite of the fact that the conflict escalates and ends in full-scale war.

For scientific, as well as applied, reasons there is an interest in a general index of an operator's efficiency. Therefore, an efficiency index derived from the quotient of individual performance and workload measures was developed. The index shows that the higher the performance in relation to mental workload, the higher the efficiency of the subjects.

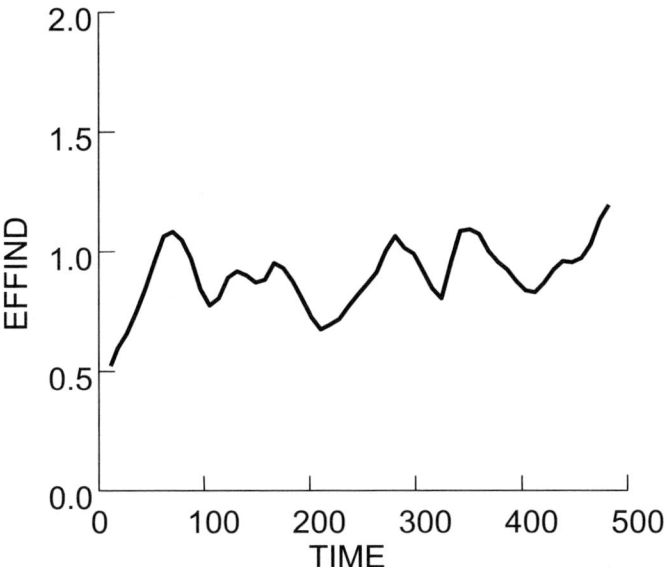

Figure 7.3   **Changes in efficiency index (Effind) as a function of time (minutes) and situational demands. The graph shows the mean trend for all operators**

Figure 7.3 illustrates changes in efficiency index as a function of time and situational demands. The curve has been smoothed by means of DWLS. As can be seen in Figure 7.3, the index of efficiency improves significantly ($r = .16$; $p = .008$) during the scenario. The operators become more and more efficient, although the scenario grows more complicated over time. The increase is particularly significant in session 1 (time between 1 and 100), session 3 (time 210–300) and session 5 (time 400–480). During session 3, the correlation between index and time of measurement is .31 ($p = .007$). For session 5, the corresponding correlation is .38 ($p = .003$). The sessions that represent different modes of escalation and war illustrate that the operators get experience and skill during these periods.

In contrast to classical experimental designs, the repeated measurement design with time series gives the possibility of presenting individual graphs or curves. Figure 7.4 illustrates changes in efficiency as a function of situational demands for each of the nine positions in the command and control group. The curves have been smoothed by DWLS.

As can be seen in Figure 7.4, the efficiency indices are in phase for several of the positions. However, it can also be observed that for some positions, the covariation is low or simply out of phase. The graphs also reveal, through their different positions, situations (of the scenario) with a higher workload than others.

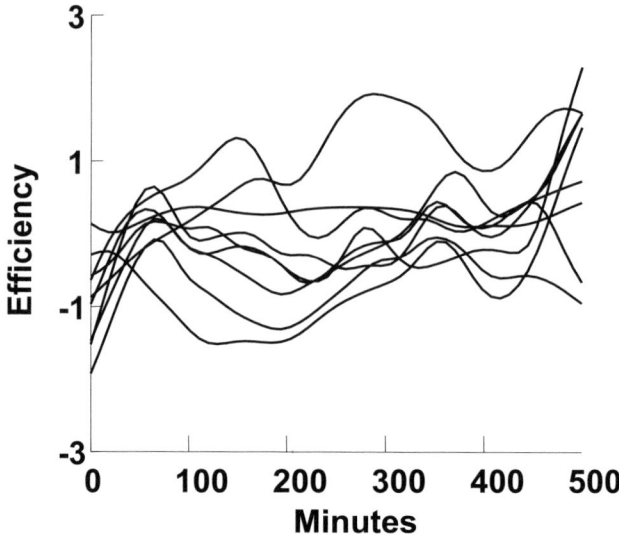

Figure 7.4   **Changes in efficiency (standardized values) as a function of time (minutes) and scenario development for each of the nine positions**

Evidently, phases of higher workload and lower performance indicate some type of functional disturbance in the total system as the positions are interdependent.

Time series bring forward information that is hardly available in/through traditional questionnaires, and their predictive potential is of special interest. The curves of Figure 7.4 are to be understood as increasing or decreasing trends of more than 30 minutes' duration. The fact that the time aspect is known means that predictions can be made and, accordingly, expected decreases in efficiency for a given position can be counteracted by different means.

By means of so called multidimensional scaling (MDS), similarities between the nine positions in regard to variations concerning mental workload can be highlighted (Hair et al. 1998). Closeness between the positions in Figure 7.5 represents the degree of similarity in individual workload profiles. Positions close to one other represent a similar workload profile (and vice versa). As seen in Figure 7.5, the positions fighter controller 1 (FSL1) and fighter allocator (CFSL) are similar, whereas the positions land component allocator (SAM) and chief current operations (CCAOC) are separated from the other positions. Significantly, marked differences can be seen between the positions SAM and track production officer 2 (MRO2), fighter controller 2 (FSL2) and CCAOC. The similarities and differences found between the positions with respect to workload reflect the content, information load and timing of the tasks performed.

Using correlation analyses, we found that there is an obvious connection between experience and performance. Relating to our data, experienced

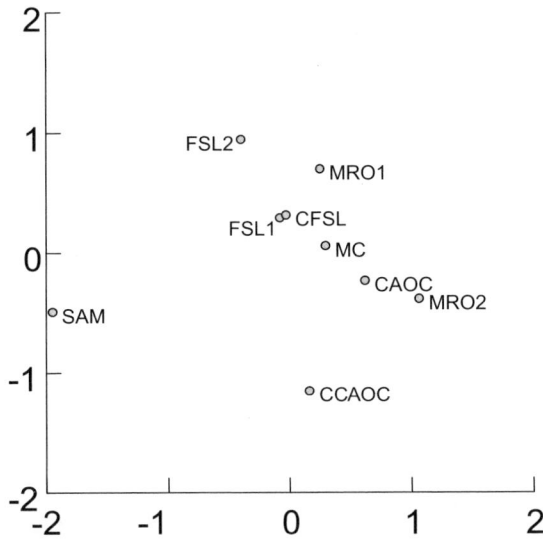

Figure 7.5   Two-dimensional presentation of similarities between different positions with respect to mental workload

operators seem to have higher performance, particularly in situations with high workload. Correlation analyses, further, show that experience, that is, time spent in the command and control system, correlates with individual as well as team performance. The degree of correlation depends on the complexity of a task. When we look at all situations in the analyses (including situations with low workload), the correlation between experience and team performance is .18 ($p = .004$). Excluding situations of low workload (PDA estimations are one or two), the relation is even stronger: .31 ($p < .001$).

Proceeding with so-called autocorrelation analyses, we found that there is a significant predictive power of workload measures performed 10 and 20 minutes before other measures (about 25 per cent of the variance of the latter can be predicted by the former). This implies that the actual workload state at a certain time can, to a great extent. predict later periods of workload and performance. The correlation plots show that workload changes form curves – even if these are based on momentary ratings. If such curves were visualized online for operators, teams and leaders of command and control operations, they would probably increase their ability to adapt – enhance – performance.

To be able to analyse the predictive power of the model in Figure 7.1, dynamic factor analysis (DFA) was carried out (see Chapter 4). The DFA is realized here by means of structural equation modelling (SEM), more specifically, using LISREL (Jöreskog and Sörbom 1993).

The terms concurrent and lagged correlations can be explained as follows. Concurrent correlations represent relationships measured at the same time.

Lagged correlations, on the other hand, represent relationships of variables measured at different times. In contrast to concurrent correlations, lagged correlations describe relationships between a certain period of time and later time periods. As an example, in our data the relation between mental workload measured 10 minutes ago and then measured again at time zero (now) represents a lagged correlation. A correlation matrix of concurrent correlations explains just what happens at a specific time. A correlation matrix of both concurrent and lagged correlations also explains what has happened, and in that respect it has a memory. This latter type of matrix forms the input to our DFA. In our study, we have scores from nine subjects on six variables repeatedly measured over three days. In all, the time series cover about 500 minutes of the scenario. First, the concurrent correlations (where lag = 0) between the six variables were calculated. Then the time series were lagged ten minutes by one measurement lag (lag = 1) on themselves and each other. This means that the variables are correlated with their own values as well as the values of the other variables on the occasion 10 minutes before. The lag procedure was then repeated for lag = 2 and lag = 3, corresponding to correlations 20 and 30 minutes before. The final input matrix was based on the Toeplitz-transformed covariances with lags = 0, 1, 2 and 3 (Wood and Brown 1994; Nesselroade and Molenaar 2004). In contrast to the concurrent, the lagged Toeplitz-correlation matrix, in our example, includes a 'memory' of 30 minutes (see Chapter 4).

Before calculating the correlation matrix, stationarity (specifically systematic trends) and distributional properties of the time series were scrutinized. A time series is stationary if there is no systematic change in mean or a trend, and if there is no systematic change in variance over time. Regression analyses indicated a modest negative trend (over the occasions) for the variables complexity and mental workload. These trends may cause exaggerated and false correlations, and, accordingly, the two variables were de-trended. (Procedures for analysis of stationarity and trends are given in Chapter 4.) To control any possible measurement error correlation over time, they were included in the LISREL model estimation (Jöreskog and Sörbom 1993).

Figure 7.6 presents the dynamics of the structural model in Figure 7.1, based on concurrent correlations between time series. The dynamic model of Figure 7.6 is also based on lagged correlations, thereby including (remembering) the relations to the time series 10, 20 and 30 minutes before.

In Figure 7.6, the manifest variables are WL (mental workload), COMP (scenario complexity), SA (situational awareness), PERF (individual performance), COOR (team coordination) and INFSH (information sharing).

The fit of the dynamic model is high, with chi-square = 281.60, df = 231, $p = 0.063$; RMSEA = 0.020; CFI = 0.99 and NFI = .99. Such a fit means that the factors and effects of the model explain the variable inter-correlations of the input matrix to a significantly high extent, if not completely.

Initiating our analysis of the dynamic model, all three factors (mental workload, individual and team performance) were set free to be able to influence later occasions.

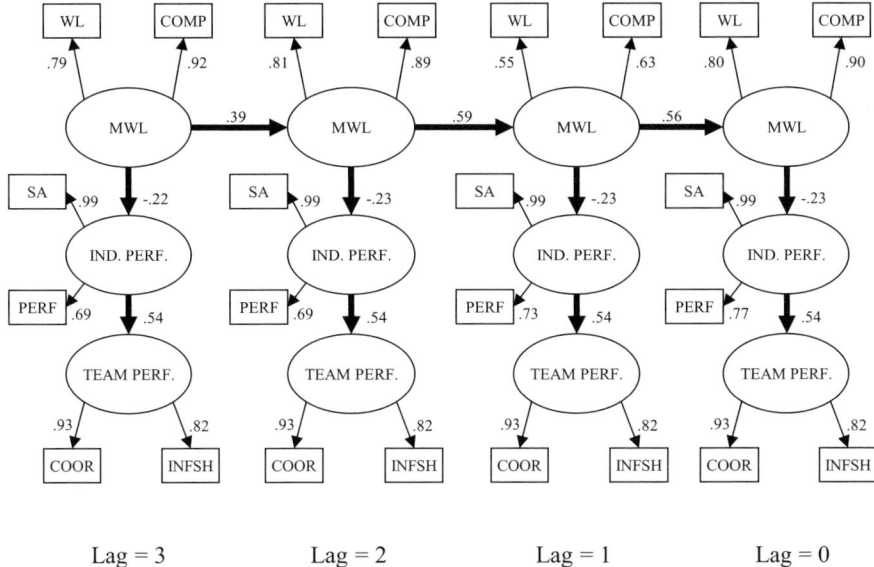

Figure 7.6   Dynamic model of the factors mental workload (MWL), individual performance (IND. PERF.) and team performance (TEAM PERF.) over three lags (30 minutes)

But, as Figure 7.6 shows, only workload influences later occasions with significance. At any given occasion (as in Figure 7.1), workload has a negative effect on individual performance and this, in turn, has a positive effect on team performance. This means that if an operator has high workload, it affects his/her individual performance negatively which, in turn, affects team performance negatively. According to Figure 7.6, only mental workload links occasions over time. Hence, mental workload has a bearing on later occasions. Our data show, for example, that there is a significant indirect effect of workload at the first occasion (lag = 3) to the third occasion (lag = 0) 30 minutes later. It is also found that mental workload at a certain occasion has significant indirect effects on individual and team performance at occasions 20 and 30 minutes later. Notably, individual and team performance at a certain occasion has no effect on performance at later occasions. An interesting aspect is that the dynamic model has a so-called simplex structure and the change process of mental workload progresses at a constant linear rate over time (Little et al. 2006; Castor 2009); simplex structures describe sequences where each factor is affected by one preceding and affects one succeeding factor.

To summarize, mental workload (variables information complexity and perceived mental workload) is a mediating factor with substantial predictive power. Mental workload can thus be used for adaptive corrections with respect to coming or arising phases of high workload and operators' reduced mental reserve capacity. To have knowledge, in advance, of coming increases in information complexity and workload can be argued to be crucial, and definitely has practical implications. For example, commanders of command and control operations can prepare, allocating resources to positions where expected increases in information may otherwise result in overload and/or decreased performance.

We have now, by means of data from CAOC in Uppsala, described how operators and teams cope with varying information load and time stress within the frames of a simulated command and control situation. Next, by means of data from the CRC in Skåne, we describe individual changes in a real situation throughout five days, 24 hours or non-stop.

In contrast to technical systems, a human operator, sometimes referred to as the human system, is affected by the circadian rhythm (over day and night), or variability with respect to vigilance, information processing, decision-making, mood and other activities and states. It is a well-known truth that human cognitive performance heavily correlates with the biological clock and that this too is reflected in circadian rhythms of heart activity, temperature and hormone levels (Monk 1991; Wilson et al. 2004).

As has been stated previously, the data collection for the second study was carried out by means of PDA systems as in the first study. However, the items were answered every 30 minutes in daytime and once an hour during the night. This made it possible to describe operators' circadian variation in terms of mental workload, situational awareness and performance.

Figure 7.7 presents the mean change in mental workload over 24 hours. The curve starts at 0830 and ends at 0800 one day and night after. The shaded area depicts evening and night (1700–0500 hours). The same area is shaded in Figures 7.8 and 7.9.

As can be seen in Figure 7.7, operators perceive a continuous increase in mental workload from about four o'clock in the afternoon until five o'clock in the morning the following day. Thereafter, the workload apparently returns to ordinary day levels. The operational experience is that the information load caused by ordinary rapid readiness operations is more or less constant over 24 hours, but this cannot explain the reported mental workload increase during night hours. Therefore, the assumed cause is probably a decrease in mental capacity (as a function of the circadian rhythm) during evening and night hours. When mental capacity, or mental resources, decrease, the relative size and importance of mental workload increase.

Few studies of the effects of circadian variations on human cognitive capacity, during operational team performance, have been carried out. However, Baranski et al. (2007), studying the effects of sleep deprivation on operational command and control performance, among other things, show that sleepiness increases and body temperature decreases at the same time as operators' mental workload increases.

Figure 7.8 illustrates how performance decreases during evening and night hours to return to day levels early in the morning. The curve has been smoothed by means of DWLS regression.

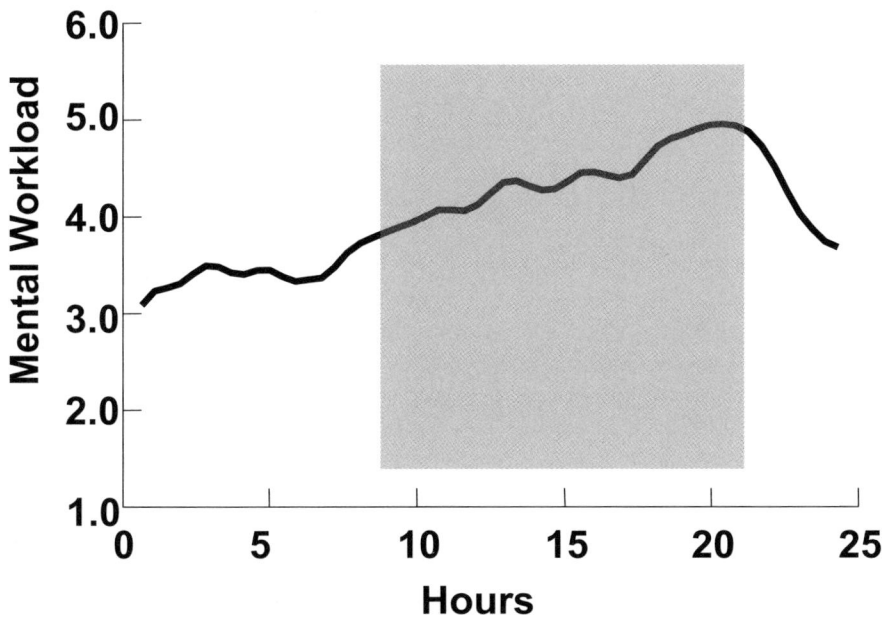

Figure 7.7   Mean changes in mental workload over 24 hours

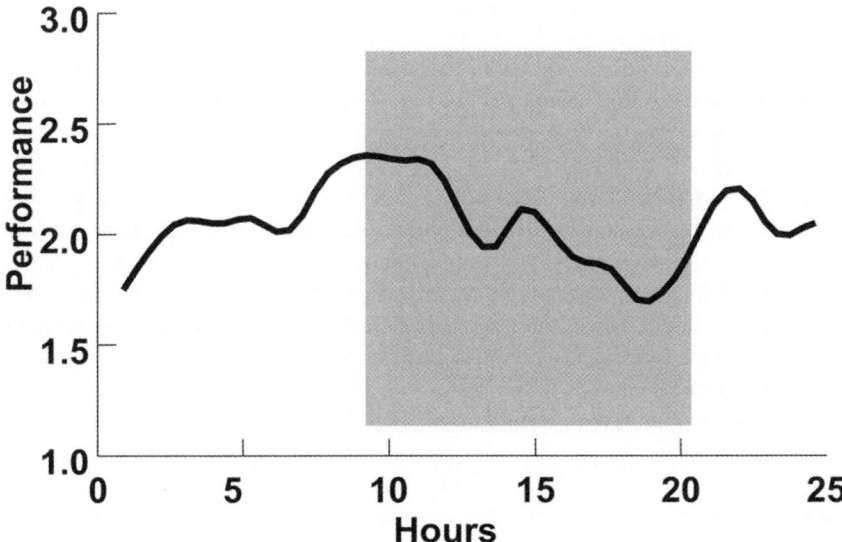

Figure 7.8   Mean changes in performance over 24 hours

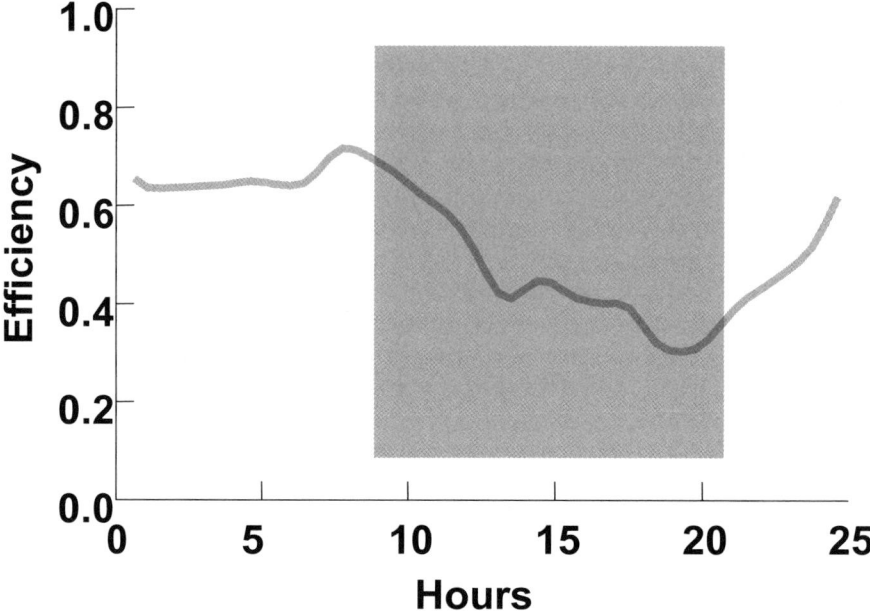

Figure 7.9   Mean changes in efficiency (performance/mental workload) over 24 hours

A comparison between Figures 7.7 and 7.8 shows that performance decreases as a result of increasing levels of mental workload. Accordingly, there is a significant decrease in the operators' efficiency during evening and night hours.

   The curve in Figure 7.9 (involving the same time aspects as Figures 7.7 and 7.8) illustrates the integrated variables' performance and mental workload in terms of an efficiency index (the same index as in Figure 7.3 of the first study). The separate trends and unique variance contributions of the two variables strengthen the validity and sensitivity of the index. As can be seen in Figure 7.9, there is apparently a marked change (impairment) with respect to operational efficiency during evening and night hours, followed by a recovery in the morning. This impairment in efficiency with a turning point in the early morning offers one explanation of the fact that accidents, on land as well as at sea, occur to a significantly greater extent during late night and early mornings.

Discussion

The human operator is a key component for command and control systems' optimal performance. Humans are good at, for example, handling complex information, experience-based decision-making and various types of situationally anchored improvisations; in addition to this, they are judicious. But compared to technical systems' performance, human performance is sensitive to external and internal influences. Human cognitive performance may be affected by, besides physical factors, changes in psychological activation and stress, circadian rhythms, information load, concentration and motivation, to mention a few examples. All these factors are likely to change over time and situation; consequently, dynamic measures of functional states, in terms of time series, can be argued to be prerequisites for knowledge and control of human efficiency.

Accurate assessments of operators' functional states are crucial for the modelling of human performance, training evaluation and implementation of decision-support tools such as adaptive aiding systems. To increase performance, safety and comfort, a system needs to 'know' the operators' activities in real time (Inagaki 2008).

The employment of dynamic measures is successful in both of the presented studies. Using PDA questions repeatedly within a scenario or a real operation (for instance every 10th or 30th minute) has proven to be a practical and functional way of measuring and understanding complex dynamic events. By means of data reduction and modelling, as it were, we comprehended the dynamics of the given scenario, and were able to describe how aspects of mental workload, situational awareness and performance interact and change over time. Out of our basic model in the first study, we could conclude that mental workload correlates negatively with individual performance, whereas individual performance correlates positively with team performance. In some sense, thus, individual performance mediates the effect workload has on team performance. If an operator has a high workload at a given moment and this affects his/her individual performance negatively, team performance will be affected too.

Structural equation modelling of relations between central aspects as mental workload, situational awareness and performance is a central Swedish issue and research area since the 1980s. By means of the technique, we could draw causal conclusions from data representing naturalistic situations of high realism and complexity. The causal relationships between workload, situational awareness and operative performance, as well as the importance of mediating factors in operational settings, have been demonstrated and verified in a series of studies (Svensson et al. 1993, 1997a; Berggren 2000; Svensson and Wilson 2002; Nählinder et al. 2004; Castor 2009; Nählinder 2009).

Time series of mental workload and performance show that during and after increases in workload, performance decreases emerge. In the same way, workload decreases are followed by performance increases. It has been noticed that a delayed and hampered performance recovery occurs when workload decreases, which can probably be explained by the hysteresis effect described by Cumming and Croft (1974). They found that the peak performance achieved during increasing demand was not reached again under decreasing demand.

Using our measurement techniques, we have been able to describe and outline training effects. We found that the efficiency index improved during a scenario even though the scenario got more complex over time. This can be explained by the fact that operators' workload decreases over time. A reasonable explanation for this development, in turn, is that operators tend to become more familiar with the scenario itself, as well as the setup, and thereby get more skilled at their tasks. This is also the case if a scenario gets more complex, for example through a higher number of war acts.

Although the efficiency index increases over time for the total group of operators, Figure 7.4 shows that there are distinct differences between several of them. By means of individual time series we obtained information about specific situations, or when different positions resulted in efficiency decrease implying a level of workload affecting the operators' performance negatively. For these situations we used the Swedish notion 'bottleneck' (in the total system's function) as the positions are interdependent.

We could also draw the conclusion that predictions can be made from the curves of Figure 7.4, and hence expected decreases in efficiency for any given position can (by different means) be counteracted.

Next, we found an apparent correlation between experience and performance, which was particularly marked during complex tasks, although already evident in situations with low workload. A plausible implication is that the importance of experience, in relation to performance, increases with the complexity of a task. So-called easy tasks require less from an operator and can therefore also be managed correctly by operators with limited experience.

Having realized autocorrelation analyses, we found significant predictive power in the workload measures. This implies that an actual workload state, at a certain time, may predict later changes in workload as well as performance. If the curves we established through analysis could be visualized online for operators, teams and leaders of command and control operations, they would be more, or better, prepared for activity adaptation and/or changes.

To be able to analyse the predictive force of the basic model in Figure 7.1, we performed a dynamic factor analysis or DFA. Even though this multivariate statistical technique is somewhat complex, it generates outcomes that can hardly be attained by other, alternative, analyses. Due to its predictive potential, DFA has so far mostly been applied within the economical sciences (Molenaar 2006).

Our initial hypothesis was that mental workload, individual and team performance would primarily influence themselves at one or two later occasions. The conclusion to be drawn from the analysis, however, was that only workload influences later occasions to a significant extent. From the basic model we know that mental workload has a negative effect on performance; from the DFA we found that mental workload links occasions over time. This means that the state of mental workload affects itself on later occasions; there is a significant indirect effect of workload at the first occasion to the third occasion 30 minutes later. It may also be inferred that workload at a certain occasion has significant indirect effects on individual and team performance at occasions 20 and 30 minutes later. Performance factors are affected by the concurrent workload, as well as workload 10, 20 and 30 minutes before. In contrast to this, individual and team performance at a certain moment has no effect on performance at later occasions.

The main conclusion we draw is that mental workload is a mediating factor of substantial predictive force. A plausible explanation is that mental workload, as compared to performance, is a state of up to half-hour trends and accordingly less influenced by short-term situational changes. Our findings thus agree with earlier research, as it is an established fact that mental workload is a key factor in regard to cognitive performance (Svensson et al. 1997a, 2002; Wilson et al. 2004). Because of its predictive potential, mental workload seems to be the principal aspect to be used for adaptive corrections with respect to coming or arising phases of high load and reduced mental reserve capacity of operators. A practical implication is that commanders of command and control operations in advance may prepare (expect) and allocate resources to positions where increases in information otherwise may result in overload, with decreased performance as one consequence.

It can be argued, or assumed, that experienced operators should know beforehand, or expect, arduous work phases and thereby be fully prepared for them. In reality, however, under high workload, operators focus and deal with momentary information, solve (acute) problems and make decisions, and are therefore less concerned with any 'derivatives' of information complexity and workload. Operators rate their workload and performance at a specific occasion – not expected changes – and they are (most probably) not aware of their previous ratings.

Our general simplex model shows that increases in information load cause decreases in situational awareness. Sooner or later, therefore, operators are affected by 'mental tunnel vision' (Easterbrook 1959). Performance is a multifaceted concept and the fewer the number of relevant aspects paid regard to, the worse the performance outcome tends to be.

As stated above, humans are sensitive to external and internal influences. One important aspect is human circadian variation in reliability and performance over day and night. This sensitivity to circadian variation makes one of several differences between human and technical systems. By means of time series data from the CRC in Skåne, we could analyse individual circadian changes in workload and performance throughout 24 hours. As compared to our study of time series data, a study based on data from a specific time of day or on data representing mean levels of workload and performance has limited explanatory power.

Interestingly, we found continuous increases in mental workload from late afternoon until early morning next day, in spite of the fact that the information load, caused by ordinary incident preparedness, was relatively constant over 24 hours.

The main cause is, obviously, changes in mental capacity and vigilance as a function of the circadian rhythm in psycho-physiological processes. When mental resources decrease during evening and night hours, the relative size and importance of mental workload tends to increase. As noted above, these findings are in accordance with those of Baranski et al. (2007), who emphasized that sleepiness increases and body temperature decreases, at the same time as operators' mental workload increases over day and night.

We identified a change, an impairment, with respect to operational efficiency during evening and night hours. The finding is in accordance with scientifically supported knowledge on the frequency of accidents on land, as well as at sea. In both cases, they are significantly higher late at night and early mornings.

The efficiency index seems to be a reliable and practical measure for capturing concurrent performance, as well as performance in the near future.

Initially, we expected that algorithms reflecting information flow and information complexity in the technical system could be used as precursor technical variables predicting the mental workload and performance of system operators. But, judging from the discussions with operational command and control subject matter experts during the planning of the study and the development of these measures, we concluded that the possibilities of developing algorithms which reflect the dynamics of information load in these systems are limited. Nevertheless, online measures of individual operator status are to be preferred, in spite of the fact that such measures may actually interfere with performance. However, the conclusion from our studies is that it did not – even if the operators, at most, had to answer the PDA questions every tenth minute.

Nevertheless, we believe that verbal communication and data link analyses (Svensson 2007) are promising alternatives to algorithms of information complexity. Successful communication is crucial for command and control performance; changes in communication patterns may, for example, indicate increases of information (for instance overload) or time stress. More generally, different types of communication analyses are windows onto team processes and explain performance factors, among other relevant qualities or contexts.

Individual operators differ as regards their experience, cognitive abilities, skill, vigilance and stress tolerance. Optimal predictions should, we argue, be based on the momentary capabilities of every single operator and this was indeed precisely the case in our studies. By means of individual predictions, operators can be optimally supported. As Wilson and Russell (2007) claim, individual predictions form vital input to adaptive aiding systems. Beyond this, individual predictions can be employed to diagnose and outline the operational status of groups or positions in command and control systems such as the command and control centres of the Swedish Air Force.

References

Angelborg-Thanderz, M. (1997). Military pilot performance – dynamic decision making in its extreme. In F. Flin, E. Salas, M. Strub and L. Martin (eds), *Decision Making Under Stress: Emerging Themes and Applications*. Aldershot: Ashgate Publishing Company, 225–32.

Baranski, J.V., Thompson, M.M. and Lichacz, F.M.J. (2007). Effects of sleep loss on team decision making: Motivational loss or motivational gain. *Human Factors*, 49, 646–60.

Berggren, P. (2000). *Situational Awareness, Mental Workload, and Pilot Performance. Relationships and Conceptual Aspects*. FOA-R-00-01438-706-SE, ISSN 1104-9154.

Berggren, P. (2005). Observing situational awareness: When differences in opinion appear. In H. Montgomery, R. Lipshitz and B. Brehmer (eds), *How Professionals Make Decisions*. Mahwah, NJ: Lawrence Erlbaum Associates, 233–41.

Castor, M. (2009). *The Use of Structural Equation Modeling to Describe the Effect of Operator Functional State on Air-to-Air Engagement Outcomes*. Linköping Studies in Science and Technology. (Dissertation.) ISBN 978-91-7393-657-6.

Cumming, R.W. and Croft, P.G. (1974). Human information processing under varying task demands. In A.T. Welford (ed.), *Man Under Stress*. London: Taylor & Francis.

Dahlström, N. and Nählinder, S. (2009). Mental workload in aircraft and simulator during basic civil aviation training. *International Journal of Aviation Psychology*, 19(4), 309–25.

Easterbrook, J.A. (1959). The effect of emotion on cue utilization and the organization of behavior. *Psychological Review*, 66, 183–201.

Essens, P., Vogelaar, A., Mylle, J., Blendell, C., Paris, C., Halpin, S. and Baranski, J. (2005). *Military Command Team Effectiveness: Model and Instrument for Assessment and Improvement*. NATO RTO Technical Report AC/323 (HFM-087), TP/59. Soesterberg, NL: TNO.

Hair, J.F., Jr., Anderson, R.E., Tatham, R.L. and Black, W.C. (1998). *Multivariate Data Analysis*. New Jersey: Prentice Hall.

Inagaki, T. (2008). Smart collaboration between humans and machines based on mutual understanding. *Annual Review in Control*, 32, 253–61.

Jöreskog, K. and Sörbom, D. (1993). *LISREL8: Structural Equation Modeling with the SIMPLIS Command Language*. Hillsdale: Lawrence Erlbaum Associates, Inc.

Klein, G. (1999). *Sources of Power: How People Make Decisions*. Cambridge, MA: MIT Press.

Klein, G., Orasanu, J., Calderwood, R. and Zsambok, C.E. (1993). *Decision Making in Action: Models and Methods*. Norwood, NJ: Ablex.

Little, T.D., Bovaird, J.A. and Slegers, D. (2006). Methods for the analysis of change. In Mroczek, D. and Little, T.D. (eds), *Handbook of Personality Development*. Mahwah, NJ: Erlbaum, 181–211.

Molenaar, P.C.M. (2006). The future of dynamic factor analysis in psychology and biomedicine. *Bulletin de la Société Des Sciences Médicales*, 2, 201–13.

Monk, T.H. (1991). *Sleep, Sleepiness, and Performance*. New York: Wiley.

Nählinder, N. (2009). *Flight Simulator Training: Assessing the Potential*. Linköping Studies in Science and Technology. (Dissertation.) ISBN 978-91-7393-658-3.

Nählinder, S. and Berggren, P. (2002). Dynamic assessment of pilot mental status. In *Proceedings of the 46th Annual Meeting of the Human Factors and Ergonomics Society*. Baltimore, Santa Monica, CA: Human Factors and Ergonomics Society.

Nählinder, S., Berggren, P. and Svensson, E. (2004). Reoccurring LISREL patterns describing mental workload, situation awareness and performance. *Proceedings of the 48th Annual Meeting of the Human Factors and Ergonomics Society*. New Orleans, LA: Human Factors and Ergonomics Society.

Nesselroade, J.A. and Molenaar, P.C.M. (2004). Applying dynamic factor analysis in behavioural and social sciences research. In D. Kaplan (ed.), *The Sage Handbook of Quantitative Methodology for the Social Sciences*. California, USA: Sage Publications Inc.

Paris, C., Banko, K., Berggren, P., Burov, A., Davis, K., Halpin, S., Kermarrec, Y., Lussier, J., Quiram, T., Schaab, B., Ward, J. and Wikberg, P. (2011). *Measuring and Analyzing Command and Control Performance Effectiveness*. NATO RTO Technical Report RTO-HFM-RTG-156. Paris: NATO.

Rencrantz, C., Lindoff, J., Andersson, J. and Svensson, E. (2007). *Evaluation of a Swedish CRC. Dynamic Measures for Performance Assessment in Complex Environments*. FOI-R-2261-SE, ISSN 1650-1942. (In Swedish; English summary.)

Silverman, D. (2001). *Interpreting Qualitative Data: Methods for Analysing Talk, Text and Interaction*. Thousand Oaks, CA/New Delhi: Sage Publications Inc.

Smith-Jentsch, K.A., Johnston, J.H. and Payne, S.C. (1998). Measuring team-related expertise in complex environments. In J.A. Cannon-Bowers and E. Salas (eds), *Making Decisions Under Stress: Implications for Individual and Team Training*. Washington DC: American Psychological Association, 61–87.

Svensson, E. (1997). Pilot mental workload and situational awareness – psychological models of the pilot. In R. Flin, E. Salas, M. Strub and L. Martin (eds), *Decision Making under Stress. Emerging Themes and Applications*. Aldershot: Ashgate Publishing Company.

Svensson, J. (2007). *Verbal Communication and Data Link Analysis*. FOI-R-2319-SE, ISSN 1650-1942.

Svensson, E. and Angelborg-Thanderz, M. (2000). Simulated landings in turbulence – Motion, predictive modelling, and psychometric aspects. *Proceedings of the AIAA Modelling and Simulation Technologies Conference*, Denver, CO. Paper number AIAA 2000-4076.

Svensson, E. and Wilson, G.F. (2002). Psychological and psychophysical models of pilot performance for systems development and mission evaluation. *The International Journal of Aviation Psychology*, 12(1), 95–110.

Svensson, E., Angelborg-Thanderz, M. and Sjöberg, L. (1993). Mission challenge, mental workload, and performance in military aviation. *Aviation, Space, and Environmental Medicine*, 64, 985–91.

Svensson, E., Angelborg-Thanderz, M., Sjöberg, L. and Olsson, S. (1997a). Information complexity: Mental workload and performance in combat aircraft. *Ergonomics*, 40, 362–80.

Svensson, E., Angelborg-Thanderz, M. and van Awermaete, J. (1997b). *Dynamic Measures of Pilot Mental Workload, Pilot Performance, and Situational Awareness*. Amsterdam, NL: VINTHEC-WP3-TR01.

Svensson, E., Rencrantz, C., Lindoff, J., Berggren, P. and Norlander, A. (2006). Dynamic measures for performance assessment in complex environments. *Proceedings of the 50th Annual Meeting of the Human Factors and Ergonomics Society*. San Francisco, CA: Human Factors and Ergonomics Society.

Wilkinson, L. (1996). *SYSTAT 6.0 for Windows: Statistics*. Chicago: SPSS Inc.

Wilson, G., Frazer, W., Beaumont, M., Grandt, M., Gundel, A., Varoneckas, G., Veltman, H., Svensson, E., Burow, A., Hockey, B., Edgar, E., Stone, H., Balkin, T., Gilliland, K., Schlegel, R.E. and van Orden, K. (2004). *Operator Functional State Assessment*. NATO RTO Technical Report RTO-HFM-056/ TG-008. Paris: NATO.

Wilson, G.F. and Russell, C.A. (2007). Performance enhancement in an uninhabited air vehicle task using psychophysiologically determined adaptive aiding. *Human Factors*, 49, 1005–18.

Wood, P. and Brown, D. (1994). The study of intraindividual differences by means of dynamic factor analysis models: Implementation, and interpretation. *Psychological Bulletin*, 116(1), 166–86.

Chapter 8

The Advance of a
Valid and Reliable Tool for
Assessing Shared Understanding

P. Berggren

Introduction

Within the command and control domain there is a need for useful, reliable and valid measures that are easy to deploy and use. The first step, for us as researchers, is to develop and test these kinds of measures. The second step is to deliver these to the practitioners and professionals working with command and control so that they can benefit from them. From the researchers' perspective there is still a lack of measures and instruments to measure sharedness. As Salas et al. (2008) point out, 'additions to the measurement approaches for capturing shared cognition constitute a significant development in team research in their own right' (p. 542).

In the area of team cognition it has been shown that there is a positive link between shared mental models and team performance (Kraiger and Wenzel 1997; Salas and Fiore 2004). Mental models are the individual's representation of tasks, systems, individuals and so on. A shared mental model is the individual team members' shared model. From experience with working with military decision-makers and command and control personnel, it is apparent that an assessment method or measure that could easily provide information about the sharedness of a team would provide useful information to commanders. There is a need for an assessment tool which can easily assess the degree of mutuality or sharedness of the mental models.

Measuring to what extent a team has a shared understanding has several benefits: for evaluation, for training purposes and for systems development. To be able to assess how well something is working, in this case to what extent a team has a shared understanding, is crucial when trying to understand why the team did what they did. For training it is important to grasp how a team develops over time, and also to capture what aspects they need to train in order to be performing together at their full potential. When it comes to systems development, it is central to understanding how operators and teams of operators function so that the systems can be designed for optimal use. A better grasp of shared understanding would provide knowledge for the systems developers to design systems that are fit for the teams using them.

The development of measures for shared understanding has been a main task since there are no measures that are easy to use, quick to deploy and can be used in theatre by officers. Our main focus has been on military lower-level tactical teams, from groups of soldiers up to the level of the company commander. These are soldiers working in conditions that have been characterized by naturalistic decision-making researchers (Klein et al. 1993) as stressful, with vague and changing goals, high risk, dynamic, complex and working under time pressure. Adding teams to this includes another level of complexity: different personal goals, levels of leadership skills, motivation, group size, training together, collocated or distributed, and so on, all factors that are likely to affect performance. On top of this, performance and efficiency are very hard to measure in these kinds of situations. Team performance is the team's results, whereas team efficiency is how well the team has functioned as a team (Essens et al. 2005, 2010).

This chapter aims at describing the process of developing measures for shared understanding. This work was performed with the goal of helping the Swedish Armed Forces get a better assessment tool for lower-level tactical team shared understanding.

Iterations of Development

The following sections will present how we have worked with, refined and developed how we look at shared understanding and how we have tried to measure the concept. This is based on six different data collections (iterations) that will be presented and discussed.

First Iteration: Student Participants

This first study was done by Berggren and Andersson (2003). The focus was on capturing how members within a team could adapt to each other. From the literature we knew that shared mental models (Rouse et al. 1992; Orasanu 1994), common ground (Clark 1992, 1996) and transactive memory (Wegner 1986) all represented disciplines and areas that took an interest in what we today call team cognition, and were also interested in explaining why teams behaved and performed as they did. Out of these theories and models we suggested two concepts that we considered measurable: overlap and calibration.

Overlap relates to the team members' representations of the team members' knowledge and abilities, and the extent to which these representations are in agreement with each other (Andersson et al. 2002). The example reads

> If person A predicts that person B will be outstanding today and if person B predicts that person B will be outstanding today, it reveals that person A and person B overlap in their predictions about person B. [p. 10, translated from Swedish]

In this case, person A and person B are in agreement about person B. Overlap is therefore a measure of how both of them understand a phenomenon; for instance, they both agree that person B will be outstanding today.

Calibration also refers to the expectations/experiences that the team members have of each other, but focuses more on an enhanced degree of understanding (Andersson et al. 2002). The example reads:

> If person A predicts that person B will be outstanding today and if person B predicts that person A will predict that person B will be outstanding today, it reveals that person A and person B are calibrated to some extent. Furthermore, if person B predicts that person B will be outstanding today and if person A predicts that person B will predict that person B will be outstanding today, it reveals that they are even more calibrated. [p. 10, translated from Swedish]

Here, person A and person B are calibrated. Like overlap, the concept of calibration is intra-team degree of agreement.

The purpose was to study how team members' degree of agreement of each other's behaviour and performance are correlated with team performance.

In this study, 120 students were used as participants, divided into teams with three members in each team (40 teams). The team were divided into two groups: friends (20 teams) and non-friends (20 teams). Friends were assumed to have higher overlap and be better calibrated since they knew each other before the study. Each friend team competed against a non-friend team in a first-person game (Operation Flashpoint) where each member controlled one game character. The objective for a team was to take out as many as possible of the opposing team's players. The participants were asked to rate their own and their teammates performance and behaviour both prior to and after the game play. Calibration and overlap were calculated from these ratings. Performance was measured using the outcome of the game.

The results did not reveal any significant findings. There was no difference between friends and non-friends either for calibration or overlap. Neither was there any effect of calibration, nor overlap, when comparing before and after game assessments. That is, overlap and calibration scores were stable over time. Friends did perform better than non-friends; that is, they won more often. It was not possible to capture the friendship effect using the measures developed (overlap and calibration). Given the definitions used for degree of agreement in this study, it was not possible to disentangle to what extent different degrees of agreement (for example overlap and calibration) were related to team performance.

The lack of association between degree of agreement and team performance might have to do with the fact that the participants were non-professionals. They were not professionally trained for the task they were asked to accomplish (they did receive training on the software). If participants had a better understanding of the requirements for each participant to carry out this type of task, they might have been better able to take each others' perspectives. One important experience with this study regarded the dependent measures: the questions regarding overlap and calibration. The participants had a hard time understanding them.

Second Iteration: Using Professionals

Reconsidering the results of the first study, professionals performing in their own domain might have been able to complete the ratings more accurately. When viewing the results in light of the theories, it could be argued that the degree of agreement among team members still might be one possibly important factor to consider in enhancing the understanding of team processes that lead to good team performance. Therefore, the next step was to study the degree of agreement in professional teams (Andersson and Berggren 2003).

The purpose of this second study was to investigate how mutual understanding between team members affected team performance. This mutual understanding was once again operationalized as overlap and calibration, only this time with professional fighter pilots as participants.

Eight fighter pilots completed 11 Beyond Visual Range (BVR) missions in a simulator (four pilots in one team competing against four pilots in the other team). Each pilot rated two items: a) all team members' performance ability (himself included) and b) how easy it was to predict each team member's behaviour during a specific mission (himself inclusive). Ratings were completed before and after each mission.

A few results were interesting, but there was no clear pattern. The overall ANOVA on overlap revealed a two-way interaction. Team outcome by period (before or after) revealed a higher overlap regarding the before ratings when winning and losing compared to equal results, and a lower overlap when winning and losing on after ratings compared to equal results. Also, teams that ended the mission with a win or an equal result had a higher degree of overlap after the mission on behaviour ratings. The opposite pattern was obtained for before ratings. For the performance question after the mission, overlap was lower for winning compared to losing, and highest for equal results. For calibration, almost the exact same pattern was revealed. Teams that *predict* individuals' performance in the same way (high overlap) seemed to perform better, but they should be less overlapped *after* the mission. For the behaviour question the opposite pattern was obtained, that is, well-performing teams should be overlapped after and not before the mission. A plausible interpretation is that the explicit rating questionnaires used were unable to capture the degree of mutual understanding, measured for instance as overlap and calibration, since the questions were difficult to understand and therefore difficult to respond to.

It was concluded that the developed instrument could not capture mutual understanding in a straightforward fashion that was easy for the participants to understand and use.

Third Iteration: Back to the Laboratory – A Microworld Study

The setback after the two initial studies halted us for a while. Yet the Swedish Armed Forces still needed to measure shared understanding, especially since a large project for developing a new command and control system was in progress. Network-centric warfare and a common operational picture was on everybody's mind. Having a common operational picture was assumed to create a shared understanding (battle awareness) of what was being planned and executed. This would in turn lead to better performance and, in the end, to winning the battle. But measuring shared understanding was still a tough question. Looking into the concept 'shared situational awareness' as an operationalization of shared understanding was another avenue to travel. Hence, in this study the focus was shifted from overlap and calibration towards the theoretical concept of shared situational awareness (Berggren et al. 2007, 2008). The main interest was still to measure to what extent members of a team were similar in their perceptions, and had a shared understanding of team goals and how to reach these goals. The lessons from the previous studies had to be adopted into the instrument, though. The questions could not be too complex or difficult for the participants to respond to. A suggested solution to this was to measure shared situational awareness using a questionnaire with predefined items that was to be rank ordered by the team members.

The purpose was to develop measures for shared situational awareness that were correlated to performance and were easy to understand and use.

Twenty-four three-member teams participated in an experiment, giving a total of 72 participants. The participants were all students from Linköping University. The microworld simulation platform C3Fire was used. This environment is mainly used in command, control and communication research and in training of team decision-making (Granlund 2003). Brehmer and Dörner (1993) characterize microworlds as dynamic, complex and opaque. Here, three participants together formed a fire-fighting team with the task of coordinating their actions in order to put out simulated forest fires. One team member controls the fire-fighting trucks, one controls water trucks and one controls fuel trucks. Water is needed for the fire-fighting trucks so that they can put out the fires, and all trucks need fuel in order to drive. Hence, there is a continuous need for the participants to communicate and coordinate their activities.

The experiment was designed with conditions using different levels of difficulty and allowing for different levels of shared situational awareness. The easier condition allowed for all participants to follow each other's actions and the development of the fire on their own operational picture. The more difficult condition did not allow for the participants to see each other's actions unless they had a vehicle located next to each other. Neither did a participant see the fire unless a vehicle was positioned near it.

To measure shared situational awareness a questionnaire with predefined items was used. These item lists were developed using a microworld subject matter expert. This preparation was intellectually demanding and costly in terms of time and effort spent. The participants' tasks were to rank the items in order of importance for the team to succeed in fighting the fires. Performance was calculated from the amount of forest that had been affected by fire. The rank-ordered items were scored using Kendall's measure of concordance (W; Kendall and Smith 1939).

There was a difference between these two conditions using performance as dependent variable. Teams performed better in the easier condition. Regarding the ranked items there was no difference between the two conditions.

These results were a bit disappointing; an experiment with a considerable number of participants had been carried out and the conditions and rank items had been developed with a microworld expert. We had tested student teams using an artificial task. Perhaps it was time to return to professionals working in their own domain.

Fourth Iteration: Moving Towards an Applied Domain

After one last attempt to measure shared understanding we regrouped and for a second time considered if the realism and motivation of professionals was called for. Consequently, the following study was done at the Swedish Armed Forces command training facility (LTA). Shared understanding is central to the commanders in a tank battalion. Coordinating and communicating within the company and with other companies is most crucial when commanding a tank company. There is a need to know where friends, enemies and non-combatants are, what is planned, what orders are issued and if some information affecting the course of action has been acquired. This was a domain where a measure of shared understanding would be appreciated.

A tank crew is composed of four members, commander, driver, shooter and loader, all with specific functions. A company commander commands 14 tanks, divided into three platoons. Company commanders and platoon leaders have dual roles: commanding the company/platoon (big picture) and commanding the tank crew (local picture). To do this the commanders have one radio network within the tank (in one ear) and the company radio network to communicate within the company (in the other ear). The company commander also needs to communicate with the battalion commander and with other company commanders in the battalion. To support the commanders the tanks are equipped with a battle management system, TCCS (Tactical Command and Control System). TCCS provides a common operational picture using a map and various symbols for information, plans, orders and the location of friendly, enemy and neutral units. The commander can send orders and plans over the TCCS to other commanders on the same network. These orders can then be clarified through verbal communication over the radio. If TCCS is shut down, the commander has to rely on memory/notes, a paper map and the radio.

The common operational picture that the commanders have is a situation picture (a representation of the current status for a specific situation), and it is a prerequisite for situational understanding. In order to be able to coordinate actions within the company the commanders need to have an understanding of what is important for the company as a team, and this understanding must be shared with the other commanders.

The purpose of this study was to test the method used previously: ranking predefined important items for the team to succeed. These item lists were developed using tank battle and tank command and control subject matter experts (SMEs). Therefore, preparing for this study was intellectually demanding and costly in terms of time and effort spent. The items in the list were carefully selected and thoroughly discussed before being included in the study. Nine officers working as tank commanders participated in this study. Performance was subjectively assessed by the participants. In each experimental run a team consisting of one company commander and two platoon leaders took part in a simulated peace-enforcing mission. All other roles within the company, and the higher commander, were performed by game control operators.

The participants considered their mental workload low, indicating that the tasks were not stressful. A higher workload would have been better as it contributes to experienced realism making participants more motivated to deal with the tasks. According to the SMEs workload would have been higher in a real-world situation. The participants judged that the teams performed well and that the team had very good shared situational awareness. Analysing the ranked items proved difficult since almost all participants ranked items almost identically. As a total, only a few items deviated among all participants' rankings. In retrospect the SMEs believed that this was because the order of the items came naturally as the tank officers had previously been trained in dealing with the situations that occurred in the study.

The conclusion was that the rank list approach had to be altered and adapted to the reality of the test situation. Preparation of the rank items took too much time and effort from subject matter experts. Also, if there was an underlying order of the items, due to training or culture, the task became too simple and straightforward. In this study, none of the participants complained about the questions being too complex or that the ranking of the items was too difficult to perform.

Fifth Iteration: Battle Management Assessment

In the previous study the participants found it quite easy to perform the rank task (to rank the items) as well as to understand how the ranked items could say something about their shared understanding of the common operational picture. Although the results did not show a relationship between the ranked items and performance, we wanted to see what happened if the order of the items was less obvious to the responders. Since the tank officers were positive about continuing the pursuit we moved on to perform the experiment in the Swedish Armed

Forces' Battalion Training Facility for tanks. The ranking of items fulfilled several of our goals with a practically useful measure: it was easy to respond to, the items was quickly ordered by the participants, it was easy to score, and results were easily comprehended. Yet the preparation time was a problem in the previous study: subject matter experts had been required to create the item lists, and it was necessary for the SMEs to have a thorough understanding of the scenario used and how it developed during game play. Therefore, in the present study, a novel approach was tested. The participants were asked to generate the items themselves and then rank each other's items. This would minimize the preparation work regarding item list development. Some experimental effort was needed to collect item lists, scramble the order of the items, and then distribute the items to the other team members. It was believed that with this approach all the benefits from the last study would be kept, while the drawbacks would be minimized.

In the present study 10 tank officers participated. The participants were divided into three teams, each team consisting of a driver, a shooter and a tank commander. Two of the commanders were also platoon leaders. The remaining commander acted as the company commander. The Swedish Armed Forces' Battalion Training Facility is a simulation facility for training with three tanks with full crew located at Skaraborg Regiment, Skövde. The tanks that are simulated are the Leopard 2. The overall scenario involved a peace-enforcing mission in a troubled area.

The experimental design involved two conditions, the same command method (all commanders used the battle management system TCCS) versus a mixed method (one of the commander's TCCS stopped working, meaning that the commander had to keep track of development using pen, paper map and notebook, doing all communication over the radio). The rankings of the items were scored using Kendall's measure of concordance (Kendall and Smith 1939). This coefficient does not say anything about to what degree the participants have a correct view of how things really are, it only represents to what extent the participants agree among themselves.

Comparing the two conditions (same battle management system vs mixed method condition) gave a significant difference using the measure of concordance as dependent variable. The degree of agreement among the participants who used the same battle management system was higher than for the participants in the mixed method condition. That is, when using the same processes and systems the commanders are more in concordance with each other and have a higher degree of shared understanding about what was important for the company to reach its objective.

There was a difference between the two conditions about how the respondents perceived the performance of the tank teams within the company. The commanders experienced that they performed better during the mixed methods condition. This was confirmed during the debriefing as well. Both participants and the observers acknowledged this, but they also made remarks that it had taken a much longer time to reach the objective while working in the mixed methods condition. That performance, in terms of consensus from the debriefing, was higher for the mixed methods condition might be explained by the fact that these teams took more time to solve their tasks and make their decisions. Yet this was discussed by the participants and observers as being problematic and as a confirmation that mixing methods and systems would degrade performance, at least in terms of speed. For tank battalions speed is an important issue, as they want the element of surprise to get the upper hand when engaging the enemy. This study has partly been presented earlier (Berggren and Johansson 2010).

Sixth Iteration: Trained Participants

Being encouraged by the results from the last study, another experiment was planned. This time the experiment was planned so that a sufficient number of teams were trained extensively on a task. Six teams with three members in each team were trained to collaborate in a microworld. The C3Fire platform was used once again. Each team member had different roles and responsibilities, controlling different types of vehicles. Every team was then trained for 10 sessions. On the 11th session the experiment was run, where the six teams put out simulated forest fires. A control group of six non-trained teams performed the same task. The experimental sessions had two conditions – easy vs difficult. In the easy condition the team members could see everything that was happening in the microworld. In the difficult condition the team members could see only what was happening around the vehicles s/he controlled. The setup was similar to the one described in the section above concerning the third iteration (see also Berggren et al. 2008). Immediately following each experimental session, the participants generated and ranked factors that they thought were important for the team to succeed. This was similar to what had been done at the Swedish Armed Forces' Battalion Training Facility for tanks, as described above in the section concerning the fifth iteration. This time the results were clear. In the easy condition the trained teams achieved significantly better than the non-trained teams on this ranked priorities measure, $F_{(1,10)} = 11.41$, $p < 0.05$. That is, the participants in the trained teams agreed more about what factors were important for successful performance, and they also agreed more about the rank order of these factors, than did the non-trained teams.

Discussion

These six studies show how we have worked towards developing a measure for shared understanding. We have moved from experiments with students as participants to professionals performing in their natural environment. We have also moved from questions that were hard to understand to rather straightforward tasks for the participants. In turn, this also led to easier analysis of the results.

The reason for moving from students to professionals was to eliminate the risk that an individual's skill affected the entire team's outcome more than the shared understanding within the team. This was a very important conclusion. In a non-professional environment, one single individual might influence the team's performance more than the other team members together. In a professional situation, each team member has a role that is better defined and therefore the team members need each other and need to understand each other to a much larger degree.

In a computer game or microworld situation the team's performance will be highly affected by individual team members' guesses of what behaviour is positively linked to performance. In our experience, the skill of one single team member in a microworld study can elevate the whole team's performance.

With professionals in real-world situations all members of the team are aware of external stakeholders' expectations. For example, firefighters work in a context where budgets, politics and real people affect, and are affected by, their performance as a team. They care not only about the current situation, but also about long-term effects on people and organizations outside the present problem. It can also be assumed that members of a professional team are working under some kind of social pressure/expectation to perform well and correctly from other team members; whether true or assumed. Thus, there is both a social pressure within the team, but also a pressure from external stakeholders.

Members of a non-professional team obviously lack this kind of pressure, especially in a situation they are not familiar with together with people they don't know very well. This can be viewed as Input–Process–Output (IPO) models with clear stakeholders, both on higher and lower hierarchical levels.

General Conclusion

Some Positive Outcomes from these Studies

An instrument that is quick to prepare, easy to deploy, easy to respond to and easy to score has been improved and tested. This is important because it will simplify the process of assessing sharedness, and it will also allow for commanders to use the instrument.

The instrument is generic, that is, the same instrument can be used in a wide variety of domains. This simplifies comparison between domains and studies.

The instrument is not limited to any specific team size; it is believed that it will work well for fairly small as well as fairly large teams. This makes the instrument more general since it does not have to be adjusted for team size. It also allows for comparison between different teams, independent of team size.

Lessons Learned

After the initial studies we concluded that the questions used (overlap and calibration) were too complex and difficult for the participants to understand. In theory the concepts might be valid, but the method of measuring these concepts was not practically useful.

Further, from a rigid experimental point of view, the number of participants was low in the studies where professionals were participating. This is a well-known challenge when working in an applied setting.

The actual outcomes in these studies are affected by many other factors apart from shared understanding. For instance, individual skill, experience, understanding of tasks and so on may all influence the outcome.

The relationship between shared understanding and performance has several other factors influencing outcome. It is possible that other factors (besides shared understanding) influence the teams' overall performance.

In order to maintain a high degree of realism and motivation we suggest that external stakeholders are incorporated into the situation, either as participants or implemented as game-controlled actors. It is believed that these external stakeholders will increase the realism of the simulation and force the participants to consider a much more complex situation.

The instrument might raise awareness of team aspects that are not normally considered. For instance, how goals are perceived and prioritized by other members can influence an individual's understanding of their knowledge. In turn, this affects how that individual adapts to the other team members.

Good teamwork is when the individuals are able to work effectively towards a common team goal. As a team matures we strongly believe that the individual team members develop an understanding for each other, their way of working, other team members' tasks and how team members might react in certain situations, and so on, thereby creating a team that can work better together. We call this shared understanding. This does not mean that there exists a shared understanding within the team, outside of the individual team members. Yet the team can be considered as a distributed entity enhancing the performance of the co-working individuals.

The instrument suggested in this chapter is a way forward in assessing a team's potential to operate efficiently. As has been shown in this chapter, there is a need for instruments and measures within the applied community; both military command and control and civil crisis response management decision-makers ask for this kind of input. Commanders would eagerly accept an instrument or a measure that they could use for assessing their own teams and staff. In this chapter we have tried to further open that door and shed some more light on these issues.

References

Andersson, J. and Berggren, P. (2003). *Team Performance: The Relation between Shared Mental Model Measures and Team Performance*. Paper presented at the Human Factors of Decision Making in Complex Systems, 8–11 September 2003. Hilton Dunblane Hydro Hotel.

Andersson, J., Berggren, P., Castor, M., Magnusson, S. and Svensson, E. (2002). *Development of an Instrument for Measuring Team Performance Potential*. Methodology Report FOI-R-0429-SE. Linköping: Command and Control Systems.

Berggren, P. and Andersson, J. (2003). *Team Performance in a Simulated Low-cost Military Environment*. Paper presented at the Human Factors of Decision Making in Complex Systems, 8–11 September 2003. Hilton Dunblane Hydro Hotel.

Berggren, P. and Johansson, B. (2010). Developing an instrument for measuring shared understanding. In S. French, B. Tomaszewski and C. Zobel (eds), *7th International Conference on Information Systems for Crisis Response and Management: Defining Crisis Management 3.0*. Seattle, WA.

Berggren, P., Alfredson, J., Andersson, J. and Granlund, R. (2008). *Assessing Shared Situational Awareness in Dynamic Situations*. NATO RTO HFM–142 Symposium. Copenhagen, Denmark.

Berggren, P., Alfredson, J., Andersson, J. and Modéer, B. (2007). *Comparing Measurements of Shared Situational Awareness in a Microworld with a Developmental Environment*. Paper presented at the IFAC-HMS 2007, 4–6 September 2007. Seoul, Korea.

Brehmer, B. and Dörner, D. (1993). Experiments with computer-simulated microworlds: Escaping both the narrow straits of the laboratory and the deep blue sea of the field study. *Computers in Human Behavior*, 9(2–3), 171–84.

Clark, H.H. (1992). *Arenas of Language*. Chicago: The University of Chicago Press.

Clark, H.H. (1996). *Using Language*. Cambridge: Cambridge University Press.

Essens, P., Vogelaar, A., Mylle, J., Baranski, J., Goodwin, G.F., Van Buskirk, W., Berggren, P. and Hof, T. (2010). *CTEF 2.0 – Assessment and Improvement of Command Team Effectiveness: Verification of Model and Instrument*. NATO RTO Technical Report TR-HFM-127.

Essens, P., Vogelaar, A., Mylle, J., Blendell, C., Paris, C., Halpin, S. and Baranski, J. (2005). *Military Command Team Effectiveness: Model and Instrument for Assessment and Improvement*. Technical Report No. AC/323(HFM-087) TP/59.

Granlund R. (2003). Monitoring experiences from command and control research with the C3Fire microworld. *Cognition, Technology and Work*, 5(3), 183–90.

Kendall, M.G. and Smith, B., Babington. (1939). The problem of *m* ranking. *Ann. Math. Statist.*, 10(3), 275–87.

Klein, G., Orasanu, J., Calderwood, R. and Zsambok, C.E. (1993). *Decision Making in Action: Models and Methods*. Norwood, NJ: Ablex.

Kraiger, K. and Wenzel, L.H. (1997). Conceptual development and empirical evaluation of measures of shared mental models as indicators of team effectiveness. In M. Brannick, T., E. Salas and C. Prince (eds), *Team Performance Assessment and Measurement: Theory, Methods, and Applications*. Mahwah, NJ: Lawrence Erlbaum Associates, Inc., 19–43.

Orasanu, J. (1994). Shared problem models and flight crew performance. In N. Johnston, N. McDonald and R. Fuller (eds), *Aviation Psychology in Practice*. Aldershot: Avebury, 255–85.

Rouse, W.B., Canon-Bowers, J.A. and Salas, E. (1992). The role of mental models in team performance in complex systems. *IEEE Transactions on Systems, Man, & Cybernetics*, 22, 1296–308.

Salas, E. and Fiore, S.M. (eds) (2004). *Team Cognition: Understanding the Factors that Drive Process and Performance*. Washington DC: American Psychological Assoc.

Salas, E., Cooke, N.J. and Rosen, M.A. (2008). On teams, teamwork, and team performance: Discoveries and developments. *Human Factors: The Journal of the Human Factors and Ergonomics Society*, 50(3), 540–47.

Wegner, D.M. (1986). Transactive memory: A contemporary analysis of the group mind. In G. Gullen and G. Goethals (eds), *Theories of Group Behaviour*. New York: Springer-Verlag, 185–208.

Chapter 9

Evaluating the Effectiveness of an Armoured Brigade Staff

P. Thunholm, P. Berggren and P. Wikberg

Introduction

This chapter presents a study of the effectiveness of an armoured brigade headquarters (HQ) in three specific respects: (a) how the HQ staff is dimensioned in relation to its tasks, (b) how staff processes work (planning, execution and coordination/decision-making) and (c) how the HQ's Standard Operating Procedure (SOP) and battle rhythm function, especially in the light of the HQ's organization and work processes. Designed as a survey study, the work is based on: (a) a military *command team effectiveness* instrument (CTEF 2.0; see Essens et al. 2008); (b) measurement of workload according to Borg's scale (Borg 1998); (c) subjective quality assessments of the brigade HQ's orders and reports and (d) verification that the brigade HQ follows its SOP. Fifty-four staff members of an armoured brigade HQ participated, facing the challenges of a peace-support/keeping operation exercise.

Results generated by the CTEF, and quality measurements on orders and reports, indicate that the HQ worked well during the entire exercise; the SOP and battle rhythm worked fairly well. However, using the CTEF, four problem areas could be identified: (a) the mission's uncertainty level, (b) high task complexity, (c) perceived instability of objectives to be attained in the mission environment, and (d) high workload level in certain staff sections. Whereas the uncertainty level, task complexity and instability of operation objectives were not under the control of the brigade HQ, the workload level could be influenced. It appears that some staff sections in the current organization are undermanned. This problem is arguably handled by an increase of some staff sections. It is also advisable to delegate duties to other sections.

Background

How effective is a specific military organization? This question is of great importance because military units are often deployed when and where there is a crisis, and lives and other substantial values are at stake. Moreover, the military, as a function, often consumes vast funds in a nation's budget, so it is important that military units are thoroughly organized and efficient. The issue of measuring the effectiveness of military organizations has for some years been a focus within the NATO research organization, and Sweden, as a partner nation, has also participated in this endeavour (Essens et al. 2008). One result of this involvement is a generic instrument for the evaluation of the effectiveness of any military team, for example, a staff unit.

In Sweden, as in many other countries, the military constantly has to refine the organization of its units in order to match changing demands from mission environments. In 2009, the Swedish Army introduced a new trial organization for the brigade staff of the Armoured Brigade Staff, and our research team was invited to evaluate this new organization in connection with a major staff exercise. We accepted this challenge and here we present how this relatively unique work was framed and conducted, thus reporting a first Swedish attempt to evaluate a brigade staff using the new NATO-developed CTEF 2.0 (Essens et al. 2010).

Our study formed part of a more extensive evaluation of the brigade HQ staff size. The new organization had a nearly 50 per cent reduction in the number of staff officers (in comparison with the previous one); this was the third exercise testing the new organization. In cooperation with the chief of the brigade staff, the purpose of our study was defined as an evaluation of the effectiveness of the armoured brigade HQ in some specific respects. Key issues were (a) how the HQ personnel (staff) was dimensioned in relation to its tasks, (b) how staff processes such as planning, execution and coordination/decision-making work and (c) how well the HQ's SOP and battle rhythm functioned in the light of the HQ's organization and work processes.

To begin with, we introduce the team concept and how this relates to a military brigade staff; further, how brigade staff activity relates to effectiveness. Thereafter, we present the fundamental CTEF model for the instrument, and also introduce measures of workload and quality as these complement the CTEF used here. After that follows a presentation of the study and its realization, results and implications.

The Team Concept

Brigade HQ, as an organization, can be regarded as a team. The team concept has been used to describe groups consisting of at least two persons pursuing the same overall objectives, interdependently of each other solving their own tasks (Baker and Salas 1997). Team members can be separated in time and space (distributed) or collocated; they can be trained together and have shared, thorough, understanding of various individuals' roles and tasks – or be temporarily arranged to solve a task (a so-called ad hoc team). It is thus a team's overall task that constitutes a team's existence. Team members can be exchanged; team size may vary over time. Using the definition above, a brigade HQ can, on a global level, be seen as a team. Looking at the brigade HQ in detail, it is more relevant to consider different sections as teams because various sections work towards different objectives, and aim to produce specific results (for example a report, or part of an order) eventually constituting the brigade HQ's 'output'. This output may, according to Brehmer (2007), be considered as the orders (produced by the brigade headquarters) issued to directly subordinated commanders (DSC), and the reports submitted to the higher command level (HC).

How can the activities of brigade HQ be understood, and how can they be connected to the concept of efficiency? A common way to describe the overall activity within an organization is to use a so called *IPO model* (referring to input, process, output), or a *transformation model*, according to which an organization processes and transforms given inputs (a military mission), and then supplies certain outputs, for example, decomposed missions to subordinate commanders in the form of operational orders (Abrahamsson and Andersen 2005; Brehmer 2007). A common way of looking at efficiency linked to the IPO model is to divide efficiency into internal and/or external efficiency (Modell et al. 2006). The internal efficiency links to an organization's effectiveness and is designed for operational performance (Abrahamsson and Andersen 2005). Internal efficiency has also been considered to concern doing things properly, 'right', while external efficiency tends to refer to external stakeholders' assessments of organizations' performance or product(s), which is, doing the right things (Drucker 1974).

Applying the concepts described above to our efficiency assessment of a brigade HQ, the aim is to assess the HQ's internal efficiency by focusing processes and organizational aspects. However, it is common that quality measurements also include ratings of customer satisfaction concerning the product that an organization produces. As customers of the brigade HQ, it is reasonable to consider the direct subordinate units, as well as the higher command, because they are the recipients of the brigade's output (orders, reports). Measurement of customer satisfaction is usually generated out of several evaluation criteria, which constitute a type of customer satisfaction index (Modell et al. 2006). Consequently, we considered the orders and reports produced by the brigade HQ as *output* needing to be evaluated to express the overall efficiency of the particular brigade HQ.

The theoretical foundation for efficiency measurements is usually organizational theory and business administration. Efficiency measures are thus often based on economic efficiency measures and therefore not easy, as it were, to automatically transfer to military organizations. Essens et al. (2005), however, developed a model and an instrument for measuring *military* command teams' efficiency. Their tool is based on an IPO model where input (prerequisites, conditions) stems from the context in which a team operates, framing what a particular team can do, and how. One part of this type of input is a team's mission. The team processes assigned to the model are either team oriented or task oriented; team-oriented factors being confidence, leadership and motivation, while task-oriented factors are, for example, information management, planning and implementation. The processes mentioned control the quality of the outcome or the team's performance, creating a division between team-related and task-related outcomes. The general idea here is that team-oriented processes control team-related outcomes, whereas task-oriented processes control task-related outcomes, although interaction naturally occurs. The model is referred to as *military command team effectiveness* (CTEF) and constitutes the model used here as the basis for evaluations of the brigade HQ. Next, a more detailed description of the model is provided.

NATO Military Command Team Effectiveness (CTEF) Model

CTEF was developed through several steps within a NATO Research and Technology Organization (RTO) project (NATO RTO HFM-085). The first step was to develop the CTEF model (presented in Figure 9.1). To evaluate the model's usefulness for command teams, a questionnaire was developed consisting of 130 items (directed at commanders and command team members), capturing the aspects and properties included in the CTEF model (Essens et al. 2005). This initial instrument was refined in 2006–2009 by another NATO RTO project (NATO RTO HFM-127), with participation from the USA, Canada, the Netherlands, Belgium and Sweden. Through case studies, factor analysis of collected data and estimates of operational relevance, the CTEF questionnaire could be reduced to 32 items in version 2.0 (Essens et al. 2010). The items were tested in military exercises (Essens et al. 2008) and in a large survey study so that they would be easy to understand and answer, while providing support for assessments of command teams at operational *and* tactical levels. At this stage of development, the results showed that, first, the CTEF model was perceived as relevant. Seventy per cent of the respondents (over 700 officers in active service from various countries) reported that the instrument addresses the main aspects of command work. Secondly, 80 per cent of the respondents considered the instrument appropriate for education, training and operations. Thirdly, it could be concluded that the term 'team' must be carefully defined *at all times* because staff members usually belong to one section while they participate in different working groups.

Turning to Figure 9.1, the CTEF model of team performance is based on a scientific, empirical and theoretical consensus that team effectiveness is a result of the main factors: *conditions, processes, outcomes* and *feedback*. The CTEF model consists of 10 components, each characterized by a number of aspects and features. These 10 components can be seen as rectangles in Figure 9.1. Examples of components are: *mission context, task-focused behaviour, task outcomes*. The features of each component are seen in the 'balloons' in Figure 9.1; for example, *situational uncertainty, managing information* and *goal achievement*. AAR stands for 'after-action review', which leads to feedback and process improvement.

The CTEF model is useful for various types of performance assessment. It is to be observed, however, that the instrument is a questionnaire, therefore not providing so-called high resolution results. The greatest advantage is that the CTEF model is validated, unlike many other similar approaches. It is reasonable that, depending on the purpose of a performance evaluation, the instrument should be combined with other measures. In this study, we used CTEF to get an idea of the brigade HQ's effectiveness. Another way of using CTEF is to get an early 'diagnosis' on a team (or several related staff units) in a command and control system. Based on such a diagnosis, a more detailed and focused plan for performance can be made, followed by organizational changes based on evaluation results. In our study, and more generally for ideas of how team members perceive their workload in the

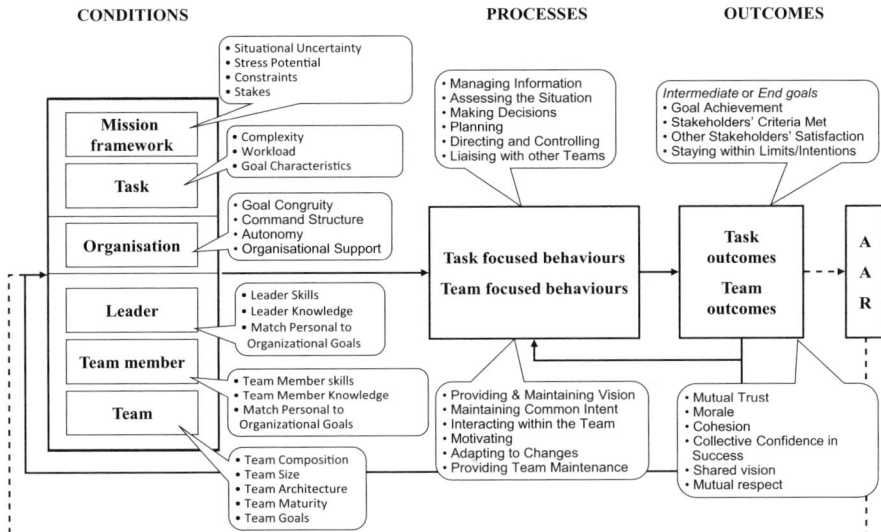

Figure 9.1   NATO Military Command Team Effectiveness (CTEF) model
Source: Essens et al. (2005). Reprinted with permission.

context of team work, we chose to supplement the CTEF with separate measurements of the team members' workload. These are introduced in the following sections.

Workload Measurement

Workload is a term that describes the effort that an individual experiences when performing a particular task; in our case staff work in a defined position. Numerous studies measuring workload indicate that the term workload is relevant and measurable *in itself*, and that it consists of several components (Hart 1986). Workload is subjectively perceived, and what is stressful for one individual need not be as stressful for another. However, the ranking of different tasks in terms of workload usually provides a good match between individuals. There are several ways of measuring how much workload an individual perceives when he or she carries out duties, for example, measurement of stress hormone secretion (Thunholm 2008a) and of emotional states using a *mood adjective checklist* (MACL; Sjöberg et al. 1979). One disadvantage with stress measurements and MACL is that these require several measurements per shift which, in turn, require interruptions several times per shift if a clear picture of the overall workload is to be attained.

The most common way to measure workload is, perhaps, to use subjective estimation employing a workload scale. *NASA task load experience* (NASA TLX; Hart 1986) is a scale frequently used. This scale is, however, less useful for the understanding of workload variance over time since NASA TLX results in estimations of workload over time sequences.

Here, we were interested in how workload fluctuates within one shift for different teams, *and* how the workload varies for different staff officers. By attaining a description of workload, we assumed that it was possible to draw conclusions concerning certain teams and specific staff officers; more specifically, finding out if their workload was too high to be sustainable over time. High, sustained workload can be an indication that an organization, or team work process, is not properly dimensioned. Against this background, we decided to measure every individual's workload throughout a shift, in the form of a subjectively experienced workload curve. This was done immediately after the shift was completed so that the interference or disruption of any individual during the shift time could be eliminated.

The scale used was based on the Borg scale (Borg 1998), a recurring tool in previous research for measuring mental effort intensity (Thunholm 2003). (For details about the questionnaire and workload measurement, see the Method section below.)

Quality Measurement

A brigade HQ leads its subordinate units through operational orders (OPORD) that may be verbal or written. OPORD, warning orders and fragmentary orders are usually in writing at the brigade level. In addition to orders to subordinate units, the brigade HQ communicates with higher headquarters, in this case a *land component command* (LCC) and subordinate units using verbal and written reports which can be scheduled (usually one per day), or initiated by a situation at hand.

In agreement with our previous discussion on *output*, we considered that the orders and reports that the brigade HQ produces (its specific output) *also* needed to be evaluated if conclusions regarding the effectiveness of the brigade HQ are to be drawn. As the brigade HQ's customers, it is reasonable to also consider subordinate units and LCC since they are the recipients of the brigade's output. The model for quality score which we designed included a number of evaluation criteria that eventually constituted a *customer satisfaction index* (see Modell et al. 2006). The criteria represent different aspects of the orders' or reports' adaptation to the recipients' perceived needs, thus reflecting the recipients' (subjective) experience of quality. The criteria, however, do not state what should be considered as somehow objectively correct; the rules for the preparation of orders and reports are assumed to govern the analyst's (or assessor's) view of what a properly designed order (or report) should look like. The criteria chosen here for evaluation have been used previously for the evaluation of military plans (Thunholm 2008b).

Study Context

The study was conducted during the last three days of an eight-day command staff exercise. To ensure that the test was to be carried out with a thoroughly trained team, only the last three days of the exercise were used; accordingly, the brigade HQ and subordinate units had established their working practices. To attain an overall picture of how the HQ had worked during the exercise, the NATO CTEF questionnaire was used, supplemented with repeated measurements of workload, brigade order quality and reports to higher command. Tracking of the staff working process was also used to ensure that the HQ followed SOP. The general assumption was that if the results from the CTEF and other measurements were good, the team was properly dimensioned and also properly organized with suitable working procedures.

To sum up, the basic idea of this approach was that we could draw conclusions regarding the brigade HQ effectiveness *if* we could expose it to a scenario where the team had to solve the tasks it was dimensioned to solve. Such an idea or study design requires a reasonably coordinated team, and also that experiment leaders can follow how the brigade HQ employs its SOP in every detail; the SOP being a template for how a team should work. If a team manages to follow its SOP when solving tasks in a realistic scenario; if its team members are not overloaded; and if the quality of the output (in the form of orders and reports) produced by the brigade HQ is good (or as planned, intended), it can be concluded that the effectiveness of the brigade HQ is good.

Method

The study was designed as a survey study, based on (a) CTEF (version 2.0; see Essens et al. 2010); (b) workload measurement according to the Borg scale (Borg 1998); (c) subjective quality assessments of the brigade HQ's orders and reports; and (d) verification that the brigade HQ applied its SOP.

Participants

The brigade HQ organization template consisted of 68 officers (including brigade commander and deputy brigade commander); four of the posts were, however, vacant. In total, 50–54 participants answered the four questionnaires. The average service length as officer (or reserve officer) was 19.6 years (SD = 9.0, min = 0, max = 34 years). As to previous experience from similar positions as during this exercise, 50 per cent of the team members were well experienced, 20 per cent had some experience, while the remaining 30 per cent had no similar previous experience prior to the exercise.

The Brigade HQ's Task

The brigade HQ's overall task for the time of the study was to engage in staff work in accordance with the brigade's SOP. The SOP includes a procedure divided into three main processes (planning, execution and decision-making/coordination). For these three processes, a standing work plan (a battle rhythm) had been defined according to when meetings and reports were due for the different processes. As a complement, there was also a detailed description of the reports that every department of brigade HQ receives from the directly subordinated units (DSUs) and sends to higher command.

Scenario

During the eight-day exercise, a scenario was run in which a multinational force was called by NATO at the request of the UN. The multinational force was assembled for peacekeeping and/or peace-enforcing operations between two nations that formerly belonged to the same federative state. The higher unit leading the brigade HQ was a land component command (LCC). The brigade HQ, in turn, led three mechanized battalions, two combat support companies and two combat service support companies. Over the three days of the exercise, the events in the scenario slowly escalated from peacekeeping to peace-enforcing activities. During the first and second days, the brigade HQ was working with planning, execution and decision-making/coordination, but on the third day no planning process took place. The scenario was familiar to the participants; the scenario events agreeing with activities that an armoured brigade should handle.

Procedure and Measurements

The CTEF questionnaire
All participants completed the CTEF questionnaire at the end of the third day. In addition to this, the brigade's planning team (an ad hoc group) completed the CTEF questionnaire once after a successful planning task; more specifically, in the afternoon of the second day. CTEF consists of 32 statements in total, and the response options are given as a five-point scale ranging from *very low* to *very high* or, for some items, *very poor* to *very well*. Sometimes, the respondents were also asked to comment on their answers if they selected any of the two most negative response options. Besides the mentioned components, the questionnaire also contained a number of questions about participants' background and experience. The questionnaire was completed digitally; the CTEF instrument was not translated to Swedish, the main reason for this being that the English in the survey is simple enough to be used by officers with English as a second language.

Assessment of workload
The exercise was divided into work shifts and, to capture how workload varied over time during a shift, the participants were asked to draw a curve on a graph where the *x*-axis represented time and the *y*-axis represented workload, expressed on a Borg scale (Borg 1998). This procedure was carried out immediately after the completion of every shift, in total three times per participant. The length of a shift could vary, but there was a link to the brigade HQ's work routine according to the SOP, including a day shift (about 08:00–20:00) and a night shift (20:00–08:00).

There was an overlap for handover between day and night shifts, extending the shifts further. The Borg scale is based on a reference value: *extremely large* (workload), that is, the heaviest workload ever experienced by the responding individual. This workload intensity was given a scale value of 13. The scale is not numeric, but based on several reference values in descending order down to *no workload*, rendering a zero scale value. The other reference points, in descending order from *extremely large*, were *very large* (numeric scale value 10), *large* (8), *moderate* (6), *low* (4) and *very low* (2). There was a possibility to draw the curve even higher than the scale value 13, *if* the respondent experienced a more intense workload than ever before. The questionnaire was completed on paper.

Assessment of brigade HQ's orders and reports
During the measurement procedure, the heads of department and staff instructors at LCC continuously assessed the quality of the brigade's reports to the LCC; this assessment took place for every report. The quality of the reports was declared in regard to four aspects: that a report (a) had the right extent and was adapted to the recipient's needs in the form of (b) resolution, (c) clarity and (d) that the report's different parts were coherent and perceived as an unambiguous message. The quality estimation was carried out as a summary score on a seven-point scale where the numeral 1 indicated very low quality, and the numeral 7 very high quality. If a score was marked as 3 or below, the evaluator was asked to supply a clarifying comment. The questionnaire was completed on paper.

Similarly, the battalion commanders were asked to assess the quality of the brigade orders and reports that they received. In addition to the criteria described above for the reports, the assessment of the orders also included commander's intent and whether the battalion commanders' task was clearly formulated.

Evaluation of the brigade HQ's status and activities
Once per shift during all three days, the heads of departments assessed the team's status and activities with regard to staffing, deviations from the battle rhythm, scheduled reporting procedures under the SOP, and the main activities that the team was engaged in. One question in this questionnaire was addressed only to the chief of staff, namely the match between the battle rhythm according to the SOP, and perceived 'actual' battle rhythm. The questionnaire was completed digitally.

Results

Evaluating the effectiveness of an armoured brigade staff is a multifaceted endeavour. The results from the various measures are presented below.

Results of the Command Team Effectiveness Instrument

When viewing the Brigade HQ as *one* team the distribution of responses is presented in Table 9.1. In the table, light-shaded values show ranges in which at least 20 per cent of the staff members chose the most positive response option. Dark-shaded values show ranges in which at least 20 per cent of the staff members chose one of the two most negative response options.

Table 9.1   Response distribution in per cent of CTEF survey for the entire brigade HQ

Item		Distribution				
		Very Low	Low	Moderate	High	Very High
CONDITIONS						
1.	Situation uncertainty is ...	1.9	22.2	53.7	16.7	5.6
2.	Goal instability is ...	1.9	33.3	44.3	20.4	
3.	Task complexity is ...		13.0	33.3	37.0	16.7
4.	Workload is ...	5.6	25.9	33.3	35.2	
6.	Clarity of command structure is ...	1.9	1.9	42.6	33.3	20.4
8.	Mix of people is ...	1.9	1.9	5.7	45.3	45.3
10.	Team maturity is ...	1.9	5.7	28.3	43.4	20.8
11.	Match of the team's own goals to the org. goals is ...		1.9	20.8	50.9	26.4
12.	Team leader competencies are ...	1.9	3.8	23.1	36.5	34.6
13.	Match of the team leader personal goals to the org. goals is ...	1.9	1.9	24.1	40.7	31.5
14.	Team member competencies are ...		1.9	18.9	49.1	30.2
PROCESSES						
17.	Decision-making is done ...		3.7	22.2	53.7	20.4
21.	Providing vision and intent is done ...		1.9	31.5	44.4	22.2
22.	Collaborating between team members is done ...	1.9	5.6	5.6	48.1	38.9
23.	Motivating is done ...		3.8	17.0	49.1	30.2
26.	Maintaining team cohesion is done ...		1.9	18.9	52.8	26.4
OUTCOMES						
28.	Staying within the limits and intentions of the mission is achieved ...		1.9	11.3	58.5	28.3
29.	Trust between team members is achieved ...	1.9		13.0	37.0	48.1
30.	Collective confidence in reaching goals is achieved ...		1.9	20.4	55.6	22.2
31.	Taking measures to improve task processes was done ...	1.9	1.9	33.3	40.7	22.2
32.	Taking measures to improve team processes was done ...		5.6	33.3	44.4	16.7

Items 1–4 in the CTEF survey have an inverted response scale compared to the other survey items. This means that the most positive responses are 'Very Low / Very Poorly' or 'Very Inappropriate' for Items 1–4. Light grey highlighted values show the items in which more than 20 per cent of the HQ members chose the most positive response option (16 of 32 items), indicating that this aspect functioned well. Values highlighted in dark grey show items where at least 20 per cent of the HQ members chose one of the two most negative response options. There are four questions

highlighted in dark grey, indicating that at least 20 per cent of the staff members perceived situation uncertainty, task complexity, goal instability and workload to be to too high. In the following we will look at these results in more detail.

The brigade HQ consists of several staff sections, and in order to get a clear picture of how each section perceived the different aspects of the CTEF the brigade HQ staff was divided into 10 separate teams and one additional temporary team for the CTEF measurement.

The following 10 teams were used: Command Group (including the Bde Cdr and composed of specialists such as Legal Advisor and Military Police); COS command group (= all Heads of Staff sections, for instance Hd G2); G2 (intelligence); G3 TOC (operations); G3 Eng (engineering); G3 Art (artillery); G3 Air (air); G4 Log (logistics); G5 (plans) and G6 (signal).

The temporarily composed 'operational planning group' (OPG = team no 11) who carried out the planning work for two days filled in the CTEF survey after a completed planning session on Day 2. The members of the OPG group participated in the CTEF survey twice. The result from the CTEF for each team is presented in Table 9.2. The teams have been numbered in the order 1–11 in accordance with the note below the table. In the table the values indicate the proportion of team members in per cent where one of the two most negative responses was chosen.

Table 9.2   Results of CTEF survey where at least 20 per cent of the team gave a negative response

Item	Team values										
	1[1)]	2	3	4	5	6	7	8	9	10	11
1. Situation uncertainty is …	80	–	–	–	33	–	25	–	–	25	29
2. Goal instability is …	100	43	22	–	–	–	25	–	50	25	–
3. Task complexity is …	–	57	67	44	–	60	25	50	50	25	–
4. Workload is …	80	43	44	33	–	80	–	–	–	25	29
5. Match of the organizational goal and the team's mission is …	–	–	–	–	–	–	25	–	–	25	–
6. Clarity of command structure is …	–	–	–	–	–	–	–	–	–	25	–
7. The support by the organization is …	–	29	–	–	33	–	–	–	–	–	–
8. Mix of people is …	–	–	–	–	–	–	–	–	–	25	–
9. Distribution of tasks and roles is …	–	–	–	–	–	–	25	–	50	–	–
10. Team maturity is …	–	–	–	–	–	40	–	–	–	25	–
11. Match of the team's own goals to the org. goals is …	–	–	–	–	–	–	–	–	–	25	–

Table 9.2   Results of CTEF survey where at least 20 per cent of the team gave a negative response (*continued*)

Item	Team values										
	1[1]	2	3	4	5	6	7	8	9	10	11
12. Team leader competencies are …	–	–	–	–	–	–	25	–	–	–	–
13. Match of the team leader personal goals to the org. goals is …	–	–	–	–	–	–	–	–	–	25	–
14. Team member competencies are …	–	–	–	–	–	–	–	–	–	25	–
15. Match of team member's personal goals to org. goals is …	–	–	–	–	–	–	–	–	–	25	–
16. Managing information is done …	–	29	22	33	–	–	–	–	–	25	–
17. Decision-making is done …	–	–	–	–	–	–	–	–	–	25	–
18. Planning is done …	–	–	22	–	–	–	–	–	–	–	–
19. Executing plans is done …	–	–	–	–	–	–	–	–	50	–	–
21. Providing vision and intent is done …	–	–	–	–	–	–	–	–	–	25	–
22. Collaborating between team members is done …	–	–	–	–	–	40	25	–	–	25	–
23. Motivating is done …	–	–	–	–	–	–	–	–	–	25	–
24. Monitoring team members' behaviours is done …	–	–	–	22	–	–	–	–	–	24	–
25. Providing back-up is done …	–	–	22	–	–	–	–	–	–	–	–
26. Maintaining team cohesion is done …	–	–	–	–	–	–	–	–	50	–	–
27. Meeting the goals of the commander and higher echelons is achieved …	–	–	–	–	–	40	–	–	–	–	–
29. Trust between team members is achieved …	–	–	–	–	–	–	–	–	–	25	–
31. Taking measures to improve task processes was done …	–	–	–	–	–	–	–	–	–	25	29
32. Taking measures to improve team processes was done …	–	–	–	–	–	–	–	–	–	25	29

Note: [1] 1 = Command Group; 2 = COS Com Group; 3 = G2; 4 = G3 TOC; 5 = G3 Eng; 6 = G3 Art; 7 = G3 Air; 8 = G4; 9 = G5; 10 = G6; 11 = OPG.

Table 9.2 presents the items where one or several teams had a proportion of over 20 per cent of members selecting one of the two most negative response options. From this it is possible to understand which teams were responsible for the negative results on the first four items of the CTEF (as presented in Table 9.1). As regards *task complexity* (Item 3) and *workload* (Item 4), eight (respectively seven) teams had several members feeling that those aspects were 'bad' (high or very high). Turning to *situation uncertainty* (Item 1) and *goal instability* (Item 2), about 50 per cent of the teams contribute to the overall negative result. Three of these areas involve the external factors, (situation uncertainty, task complexity and goal instability). These are, indeed, aspects that the brigade HQ does not control. One area that *can* be controlled by the brigade HQ's organization and working procedures, on the contrary, is individual staff members' workload. The two teams where 80 per cent considered themselves as having a high workload are Command Group and G3 Art (see Table 9.2). In a way, this makes sense because the Command Group included several *one-person functions*; G3 Art had been working with labour-intensive processes, such as targeting or combined effects working group. For all other areas included in the CTEF, besides the four mentioned above, it was clearly less than half, usually 1–3 teams per item, which had more than 20 per cent of members who responded negatively.

As regards *information management* (Item 16), four teams had a relatively high proportion of negative responses. Interestingly, one of these teams was COS Command Group, that is, the team to which all section heads belonged. One team (G6) differed from the other teams by perceiving relatively many areas negatively (as shown by more than 20 per cent of the team members).

The questions where more than 20 per cent of the team members chose the most positive response option on CTEF are presented in Table 9.3. In the table, the values indicate the proportion of team members in per cent where the most positive response was chosen.

Table 9.3   Results of the CTEF survey where at least 20 per cent of the team chose the most positive response option

Question	Team values										
	1[1]	2	3	4	5	6	7	8	9	10	11
4. Workload is …	–	–	–	22	–	–	–	–	–	–	–
5. Match of the organizational goal and the team's mission is …	–	–	–	–	33	–	25	–	–	25	29
6. Clarity of command structure is …	60	43	–	–	–	–	–	33	–	50	29
7. The support by the organization is …	–	–	–	–	–	40	–	–	–	–	–
8. Mix of people is …	100	57	33	33	67	40	–	80	–	25	43
9. Distribution of tasks and roles is …	60	43	–	–	–	40	25	33	–	–	–
10. Team maturity is …	–	29	22	–	–	40	–	40	–	25	–
11. Match of the team's own goals to the org. goals is …	60	43	25	–	33	40	–	–	–	25	–
12. Team leader competencies are …	100	43	22	22	33	40	–	60	–	–	–
13. Match of the team leader personal goals to the org. goals is …	60	29	22	–	67	–	25	50	50	25	–
14. Team member competencies are …	100	29	33	33	–	–	–	40	–	–	29
15. Match of team member's personal goals to org. goals is …	60	–	–	–	–	60	–	33	–	–	–
16. Managing information is done …	40	–	–	–	–	–	25	–	–	–	–
17. Decision-making is done …	80	–	–	–	67	–	25	–	50	25	–
18. Planning is done …	80	–	–	–	–	–	–	–	–	–	–
19. Executing plans is done …	80	–	–	–	33	40	25	–	–	–	–
20. Interacting with other command teams is done …	80	29	–	22	33	–	50	–	–	–	–
21. Providing vision and intent is done …	80	–	–	22	67	–	–	–	–	25	–
22. Collaborating between team members is done …	60	29	44	44	33	40	25	50	50	–	29
23. Motivating is done …	60	43	22	22	–	–	–	80	–	25	–
24. Monitoring team members' behaviours is done …	40	–	22	–	–	–	33	33	–	–	–

	1	2	3	4	5	6	7	8	9	10	11
25. Providing back-up is done …	60	–	–	–	–	–	–	–	–	–	–
26. Maintaining team cohesion is done …	80	29	–	22	33	–	50	–	50	33	–
27. Meeting the goals of the commander and higher echelons is achieved …	60	–	–	–	33	–	25	–	–	25	–
28. Staying within the limits and intentions of the mission is achieved …	80	–	–	22	67	–	25	33	–	50	–
29. Trust between team members is achieved …	100	43	33	56	–	–	25	83	50	50	–
30. Collective confidence in reaching goals is achieved …	80	–	–	22	33	–	–	50	–	–	–
31. Taking measures to improve task processes was done…	40	43	22	33	–	–	–	33	–	–	–
32. Taking measures to improve team processes was done …	–	–	33	22	–	–	–	33	–	–	–

Note: [1)] 1 = Command Group; 2 = COS Com Group; 3 = G2; 4 = G3 TOC; 5 = G3 Eng; 6 = G3 Art; 7 = G3 Air; 8 = G4; 9 = G5; 10 = G6; 11 = OPG.

The CTEF results in Table 9.3 indicate that there are numerous areas where several teams have a higher percentage of positive responses (more than 20 per cent of the team members chose the most positive response option). For 10 of the 32 items, more than 50 per cent of the teams had a high proportion of positive team members.

The most positive areas appeared to be team composition and collaboration between team members; also trust between team members, and the assessment that the team leader's personal goals were consistent with the organization's goals, are manifested as highly positive. The team which had the highest percentage of positive team members (concerning the largest number of item areas) was the Command team. To summarize the results, the brigade HQ generally accomplished positive responses on the CTEF survey.

Workload Measurements Results

The work shifts had an average length of just about 15 hours (M = 14.6, SD = 2.3). To some extent, the standard deviation depends on the fact that some participants left the exercise in advance. The work shift length was otherwise stable at about 15 hours.

The average maximum value on the workload scale reported by the team members during a shift was M = 7.4 (SD = 2.5), where 'very high' workload had the value 10 and 'very low' workload matched the value 2. The average of the minimum value reported by the team members was M = 3.0 (SD = 2.2). The difference between individual participants' highest and lowest reported value was M = 4.0 (SD = 2.6). The average figures indicate that the workload on average over a shift ranged roughly between 'low' and 'high'. Taking into account also the standard deviation, it can be concluded that a certain proportion of HQ members at least occasionally also had 'very high' workload; some occasionally a 'very low' one.

In summary, the workload measurements varied within and between teams, and also between different days. Considering the regular activities of the brigade HQ during the various days, the variation makes sense. For example, the total workload was less intense the third day because no long-term planning and work on orders remained. This was particularly evident for section G5, which during the first two days reported that the maximum workload was 'high', while it was closer to 'very low' the third and last day. The results also show that certain sections had their constant average maximum load at a reasonably high value, between 'moderate' and 'very high', while the difference between the highest and lowest values was relatively small. This was particularly true for the TOC and G9. It is also obvious that there was consistency between the CTEF measurement of workload and the Borg scale, which is a more specific and detailed tool for workload measurement. Both analytic instruments indicated that the G3 Art and the Command Team involved several officers experiencing high workload; incidentally, this is also the case for G9. The workload survey showed that G3 Art and Command Team were busy mainly on the days when comprehensive planning *and* execution went on.

Results Concerning the Quality of Orders and Reports

The assessment of the quality of reports and orders indicates that the quality was reasonably high for reports submitted to the LCC (M = 4.8; n = 18, SD = 1.5, min = 1, max = 7) and high for the reports issued to the DSU (M = 5.9; n = 7, SD = 0.9, min = 5, max = 7). The assessment of written orders issued to the DSU indicates a reasonably high quality (M = 5.2; n = 6, SD = 1.7, min = 3, max = 7). Comments from the raters on the orders/reports which received a lower rating than 3 were few, and mainly in the categories wrong content (too much extraneous text but also in some cases too few report areas included), and a lack of adaptation towards the recipient's need for level of detail (too little detail in an intelligence report).

One conclusion is that the brigade HQ produced, published, reports and orders of good quality, with few exceptions. Averages around 5 on a 7-point rating scale can be considered a good rating and indicate that a product essentially meets a customer's needs and expectations.

Results from the Evaluation of Brigade HQ Status and Activities

In the survey that was returned once per day by the section heads, only one section reported that vacancies in that section had affected the section's overall ability to function; the G4 lacked a chief technical officer, a communications officer and a logistics officer for part of the time. This implied that these functions were not active during the exercise. Another reported deviation regarding personnel was that the position of deputy brigade commander was vacant.

As to deviations from the SOP and battle rhythm, the brigade HQ constitutes a marked case concerning the number of reports sent to the LCC; only 50 per cent of the regular reports included in the SOP were sent every day. Apart from that, section heads reported only minor, temporary deviations. On the issue of whether the activities carried out could be described as normal business for the section, all section heads at all times reported agreement.

In addition to the deviations reported by the section heads, a number of other factors were considered to have affected the evaluation of the brigade HQ. First, the brigade HQ was deployed in an indoor location during the entire exercise. Second, the brigade HQ worked during extended day shifts, complemented with reduced night shifts (reduced TOC). This in itself need not be unrealistic, but it does mean that the team's endurance (in more intensive operations) has not yet been tested. Third, there were no other operative units participating in the exercise (except for the brigade HQ), and that reduced the information flow to HQ and prevented the consequences of faulty decisions or delays; it also simplified the interaction and visits to other command posts. Fourth, there was no increase in stress due to real danger or to morally or ethically difficult decisions that had to be taken. Fifth, the brigade HQ had less than 100 per cent manning, which need not be unrealistic as the manning of the staff nevertheless was relatively high. Sixth, all functions were not fully represented in the scenario; the section heads mentioning such deficiencies belonged to G1, G2, G3 Art and G4. Lastly, the information management system was not used as initially intended for collaboration within the staff (according to head of the G3 TOC).

Realism of the Exercise

To understand the results of the evaluation of the HQ it was necessary to investigate whether the exercise was perceived as sufficiently realistic or not. One statement posed to the participants for them to agree or disagree with was: 'The latter part of the exercise has provided sufficiently realistic conditions in order to be able to form an opinion regarding the brigade HQ's ability to solve its tasks in a realistic field environment.' This statement complemented the CTEF survey and responses were given on a five-step scale (numerals denoting: 1 = strongly disagree; 3 = partly agree, partly disagree; and 5 = strongly agree).

The brigade HQ's response distribution, as a whole, indicates that a majority of the participants (28) selected response option 1 or 2 and therefore did not support that the exercise provided sufficiently realistic conditions to be able to form a reasonable opinion of the brigade HQ's ability to solve their tasks in a real-world situation. Other participants (14) chose option 3 (no set view), while only 12 participants were positive that the exercise was realistic enough to permit evaluation of the brigade HQ organization and work processes, an experience we return to in the next section.

Discussion

The purpose of this study was to evaluate the effectiveness of an armoured brigade HQ in some specific respects. Key issues were (a) how the HQ personnel (staff) was dimensioned in relation to its tasks, (b) how staff processes such as planning, execution and coordination/decision-making work, and (c) how well the HQ's SOP and battle rhythm functioned in the light of the HQ's organization and work processes. For this we employed the CTEF, completed with measurements of workload and quality of orders and reports issued by the brigade HQ.

The overall result of the CTEF and the quality measurements of orders and reports indicate that the brigade HQ worked well during the exercise. Of the four areas that team members found troubling, three are not expected to be influenced to a significant extent by the way in which the brigade HQ is organized. The fourth and only area which actually could be influenced is *workload*; a phenomenon momentarily heavy or even very heavy for some officers, while lower for others. No team member risked being exhausted since the work schedule of the HQ permitted rest for at least 6–9 hours between shifts (which were a maximum of 15 hours).

There were no findings (save for a few comments) suggesting that the brigade HQ's three working processes and SOP did not work. However, it was evident that when all three processes were ongoing (in parallel), the workload was relatively high, putting demands on the particular functions that were organizationally short of personnel. Redundancy in one of the brigade's departments (G9) was low with the current organization and work procedure. The conclusion, thus, is that the brigade HQ worked well even if it seems probable that (with the present organization and task division) the Civil–Military collaboration (CIMIC) function (G9) risks quickly becoming an obstruction for the HQ. It remains to be explored how the information management of the HQ can be improved. The CTEF evaluation made it clear that one of the sections (G6) was significantly more negative concerning several CTEF items in comparison with other sections. Further investigations are thus also needed on this point.

To what extent may we generalize all these findings to a real-world mission involving the brigade HQ? Considering the results from the exercise's realism (last in the Results section), it seems reasonable not to generalize the resulting outcomes. The main reason for this is that this exercise did not, to a significant extent, provide a fully realistic environment. Any wider, more general, conclusions about the brigade HQ's staffing, or the dimensions of the sections, must therefore be constrained. There was a lack of real subordinate units; several actual functions were not included; and most of the exercise was carried out in a low-intensity scenario, so we refrain from inferring whether the brigade HQ was properly dimensioned in size or not. Still, there is no apparent reason why the brigade HQ's processes and procedures (SOPs) would not work in a real situation. The workload will, of course, gradually increase, but so do the team members' energy and motivation. In a regular peacekeeping or peace-enforcing mission, team members quickly learn and manage routines. Albeit the HQ's dimension for a high-intensity conflict has not been tested during this exercise, the HQ is (with its present SOP) not designed to work non-stop with all functions fully manned.

Before any further, detailed evaluation can be made, it is necessary to identify and address weaknesses thoroughly. For example, the SOP needs to be a bit clearer in regard to which reports are to be used at all, which to remain verbal and, again, which reports need to progress within the organization (to DSUs). Another matter needing clarification in the SOP is how different HQ staff alert levels should be translated into manning and the readiness of members of different staff sections. Manning and work procedures within the section that were identified as having very high workload need to be reviewed. It would also be useful to investigate whether there are any potential flaws in the HQ information management process.

If a future objective is to evaluate the manning of the brigade HQ (being difficult to draw general conclusions on this issue here), the next evaluation should arguably be implemented in a more pronounced high-conflict scenario with more intensive non-stop operations. It is also desirable to have more complete manning of the functions of the brigade HQ's recipients, specifically Higher HQ and DSUs, and not only small cadre units. Our assessment is that the improvements in these areas are necessary to test the brigade HQ's manning dimension.

A structured follow-up of the brigade HQ could continue along the same lines as followed in this evaluation. Such an evaluation should focus on both achieving a more intense and complete scenario around the brigade HQ, so that the manning dimension can be tested, and also following up on suggested changes in the SOP as a result of the findings from this evaluation.

Finally, we also want to add that this evaluation was presented to the brigade staff and perceived to be helpful and of value for the continuing development of the brigade HQ. This resulted in a prolonged collaboration between our team and the Swedish Armed Forces, for which we have further developed and tested a Swedish version of the CTEF.

References

Abrahamsson, B. and Andersen, J.A. (2005). *Organisation – att beskriva och förstå organisationer*, tredje uppl. Malmö: Liber Ekonomi.

Baker, D.P. and Salas, E. (1997). Principles for measuring teamwork: A summary and look toward the future. In M. Brannick, E. Salas and C. Prince (eds), *Team Performance Assessment and Measurement: Theory, Methods, and Applications*. Mahwah, NJ: Lawrence Erlbaum Associates, Inc., 331–55.

Borg, G. (1998). *Borg's Perceived Exertion and Pain Scales*. Champaign, IL: Human Kinetics.

Brehmer, B. (2007) *Vad är Ledningsvetenskap?* Kungl. Krigsvetenskapsakademiens Handlingar och Tidskrift.

Drucker, P.F. (1974). *Management: Tasks, Responsibilities, Practices*. New York: Harper & Row.

Essens, P., Vogelaar, A., Baranski, J., Berggren, P., van Buskirk, W., Goodwin, G.F. and Mylle, J. (2008). *Measuring Command Team Effectiveness*. Paper presented at the HFM-142 Symposium on Adaptability in Coalition Teamwork, 21–23 April 2008. Copenhagen, Denmark.

Essens, P., Vogelaar, A., Mylle, J., Baranski, J., Goodwin, G.F., Van Buskirk, W., Berggren, P. and Hof, T. (2010). *CTEF 2.0 – Assessment and Improvement of Command Team Effectiveness: Verification of Model and Instrument*. NATO RTO Technical Report TR-HFM-127.

Essens, P., Vogelaar, A., Mylle, J., Blendell, C., Paris, C., Halpin, S. and Baranski, J. (2005). *Military Command Team Effectiveness: Model and Instrument for Assessment and Improvement*. Technical Report AC/323(HFM-087)TP/59.

Hart, S.G. (1986). Theory and measurement of human workload. In J. Zeidner (ed.), *Human Productivity Enhancement*. New York: Praeger, 496–555.

Modell, S., Grönlund, A., Wiesel, F., Wittbom, E. and Norlander, N.-O. (2006). *Effektivitet och styrning i statliga myndigheter*. Lund: Studentlitteratur.

Sjöberg, L., Svensson, E. and Persson, L.-O. (1979). The measurement of mood. *Scandinavian Journal of Psychology*, 20(1), 1–18.

Thunholm, P. (2003). Military decision making under time-pressure: To evaluate or not evaluate three options before the decision is made? In P. Thunholm, *Military Decision Making and Planning: Towards a New Prescriptive Model*. Doctoral dissertation at Stockholm University. Edsbruk: Akademitryck.

Thunholm, P. (2008a). Decision-making styles and physiological correlates of negative stress: Is there a relation? *Scandinavian Journal of Psychology*, 49, 213–19.

Thunholm, P. (2008b) Providing battlespace information to reduce uncertainty: Will more information lead to better plans? *Journal of Cognitive Engineering & Decision Making*, 2(4), Winter, 295–310.

Chapter 10

Organizational Effectiveness at the Kosovo Force Headquarters: A Case Study

M. Granåsen and J. Marklund

Introduction

In describing the methods and results of the case study that was performed by NATO HFM-163, *Improving the Organisational Effectiveness of Coalition Operations*, at the KFOR headquarters (HQ) in Pristina (Kosovo) in 2010, the purpose of this chapter is twofold. First, it demonstrates how organizational effectiveness can be assessed in an operative multinational environment. Second, it shows some of the benefits from a single research organization's participation in a multinational research constellation such as that within the NATO Research and Technology Organisation (RTO) programme. In this introductory section, the NATO RTO is described and the usefulness of programme participation is discussed. Thereafter follows a description of the work that has been carried out by the HFM-163 research group, including a brief description of a theoretical model for organizational effectiveness that this group has developed. Research group 163 is organized under the NATO RTO Human Factors and Medicine panel; hence its reference is HFM-163. The remaining chapter describes the Kosovo case study, which was conducted as an attempt to validate the model.

On Participation in a Multinational Research Programme

The NATO RTO promotes and conducts cooperative scientific research across, and exchanges information with, a total of 28 NATO nations and 38 NATO partners – see the NATO RTO (2011) webpage. This implies that RTO encompasses over 3,000 scientists and engineers, all addressing a wide scope of defence technologies and operational domains. This effort is supported by an executive agency, the Research and Technology Agency (RTA), which facilitates the collaboration by organizing a wide range of studies, workshops and symposia, as well as other forums in which researchers can meet and exchange knowledge. The RTO is led by the Research and Technology Board (RTB), constituted by up to three leading authorities (persons) in defence research and technology from every NATO nation.

There are a total of eight main panels within the RTO, all having different focuses and aims. One of these panels is the HFM panel which is the focus for the present work. The mission for the HFM panel is to provide the science and technology base for optimizing health, human protection and wellbeing, and human performance in operational environments. This involves understanding of and guarantees for physical, physiological, psychological and cognitive compatibility among military personnel, technological systems, missions and environments.

The Swedish Defence Research Agency (FOI) only commits to groups that focus research areas of particular interest for Sweden, that is, for FOI and/or the Swedish Armed Forces. This means that participation in such research groups constitutes a unique opportunity to work with distinguished researchers from different countries. By combining the research efforts of a number of different countries, the group can achieve much more than a single nation would be able to do during the same time. Since the aim of the groups is to optimize performance for humans in operational environments, research results are usually of direct use for the Swedish Armed Forces and FOI. The next section will describe the work of the NATO HFM research group number 163, more specifically that which has hitherto been referred to as *Improving the Organisational Effectiveness of Coalition*.

NATO Research Group

NATO HFM-163 (*Improving the Organisational Effectiveness of Coalition Operations*) is a research group initiated in 2007 (and discontinued in 2011). During this time, the group was composed of members from 15 NATO and Partnership for Peace (PfP) countries. All participating countries had one or two representatives in the group. Sweden contributed two researchers throughout the given term.

The purpose of the group's research was to improve organizational effectiveness, thus improving work in multinational coalitions, with particular focus on the organizational effectiveness of a multinational military headquarters (operational level).

Between 2007 and 2009, the group focused on literature reviews, interviews with subject matter experts (SMEs) and focused discussion groups to develop a model for organizational effectiveness. There are several ways of approaching organizational effectiveness; for example, from an internal resource approach, an external resource approach or a technical approach. As regards the internal approach, one looks at the innovation potential as well as functional aspects, such as the ability to be quick and responsive. The external resource approach, on the other hand, focuses the ability to secure, manage and control key skills and resources. Thirdly, the technical approach to organizational effectiveness concerns the ability to efficiently convert skills and resources into goods and services (Daft 1998).

After a comprehensive literature review, the HFM-163 group decided to study organizational effectiveness from an internal resources approach. According to this, effectiveness is assessed by indicators of internal conditions and efficiency, such as efficient use of resources and harmonious coordination between departments. Goals are created by the management of the organization against which effectiveness can be assessed. Jones (2004) describes two types of goals that can be used to evaluate organizational effectiveness: official goals and operative goals. *Official goals* are an organization's guiding principles, usually formally stated in its annual report and in other public documents. *Operative goals* are long- and short-term goals that, so to say, put management and employees on the right track when they perform organizational work. Examples of operative goals are, for example, reduced decision-making time, increased motivation of employees or reduced conflict between organization members (Jones 2004).

To decide exactly which indicators and goals are appropriate to use for the assessment of organizational effectiveness in a NATO HQ, four organizational effectiveness models were analysed in detail: (a) the Command Team Effectiveness Model (CTEF; Essens et al. 2005), (b) the star model (Galbraith 2002), (c) the 7-S model (Peters and Waterman 1982), and (d) the Behavioural Engineering Model (BEM; Gilbert 1996). The different models can be argued to have strengths and weaknesses; to some extent, they also cover different aspects of organizational effectiveness. After analysing and comparing the models, the group decided to develop a new model, using the aspects that were deemed most relevant and applicable to the effectiveness of coalition HQs.

The HFM-163 Organizational Effectiveness Model

The HFM-163 group created a model consisting of three parts: *input factors*, *operative goals* and *official goals*. Based on the literature review and discussions with SMEs, the group came to the conclusion that both operative goals and official goals need to be considered in assessing the organizational effectiveness of a NATO HQ. The group decided to make the following assumption. The main official goal of a NATO coalition HQ staff is to support the troops on the ground in conducting their operation, that is, to provide effective command and control. This assumption can be argued to be fulfilled when three operative goals are achieved: (a) effective and timely sharing of information, (b) effective and timely decision-making and (c) improved shared awareness of tasks and responsibilities. Previous research on organizational effectiveness has revealed that structure, people, processes and culture must be *aligned* towards these operative goals if the main goal is to be reached effectively (Porter 1996). Consequently, the model stipulates that NATO HQs have to make sure that the decisions made concerning the NATO HQ's structure, processes, people and culture support the accomplishment of the operative goals. Figure 10.1 shows this hypothesized process. Following Figure 10.1, the different components of the model are explained in detail.

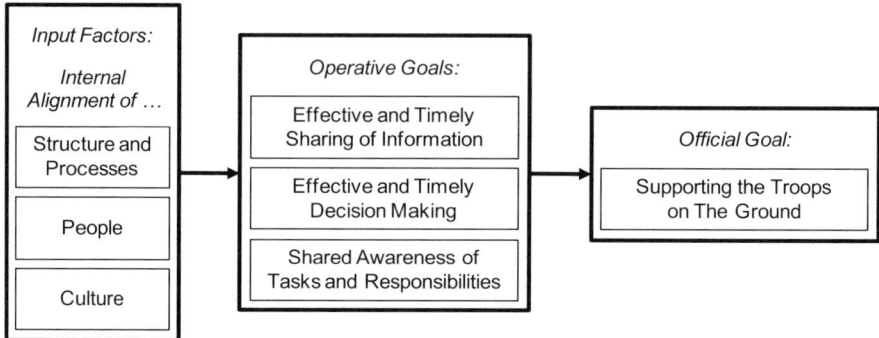

Figure 10.1   Model of organizational effectiveness of so-called Non-Article 5 Crisis Response Operations HQ

Operative goals
Effective and timely sharing of information concerns the way the HQ handles information or knowledge, that is, its effectiveness depends on how well the HQ can acquire and manage information. Three features of information sharing are important: (a) obtaining, (b) processing and (c) exchanging information (Essens et al. 2005). *Effective and timely decision-making* includes (a) identifying or creating multiple options, (b) choosing among alternatives by integrating the differing perspectives and opinions of team members, (c) implementing optimal solutions and (d) monitoring the consequences of these solutions. The effectiveness of an HQ's decisions lies in their quality, timeliness and efficiency (Essens et al. 2005). *Shared awareness of tasks and responsibilities* concerns the understanding of what different members of the organization are doing to get a common understanding of their different roles and responsibilities. The assumption is that unless the HQ can ensure a clear, accurate and common understanding of those duties, its organizational effectiveness may be compromised.

Input factors
Structures and processes constitutes an input factor, where *structure* refers to the formal system of task and authority that controls how people act and use resources to achieve organizational goals (Jones 2004), and *processes* refers to the way an organization implements its objectives in the organizational structure at hand (Peters and Waterman 1982). HFM-163 presumes that structure needs to be aligned with processes, so that when the structure is 'flat', then processes should be decentralized, if the organization is to reach their operative goals of effective and timely information sharing, decision-making and shared awareness of tasks and responsibilities. Furthermore, the research group expects that the greater the degree to which the NATO HQ's organizational structure and processes resemble those of an *organic organization*, the more likely it is that these factors will support the accomplishment of operative goals. Organizations with an organic

organizational structure are *decentralized* (which means that the authority to make important decisions resides at all levels in the hierarchy), stimulates *flexibility* (so employees can innovate, adapt to changes and make decisions when necessary) and *roles are loosely defined* (that is, organizational members with different functions work together to solve problems).

These structural and process factors are also closely linked to the factors people and culture. The input factor *people* concerns how leadership is executed. The HFM-163 group presumes that the leadership should be transformational, that is, the leaders should behave in the way they want their subordinates to behave (idealized influence); they should motivate and inspire their followers (inspirational motivation); they should encourage creativity and new approaches (intellectual stimulation) and they should pay special attention to every individual's need for achievement and growth by acting as coach and mentor (individualized consideration).

The input factor *culture* encompasses both organizational and national culture. Both aspects could be important in a NATO HQ, but the HFM-163 group focuses primarily on organizational culture as this phenomenon more specifically addresses the values and work practices of a NATO HQ. An organization's culture consists of the end states that the organization wants to accomplish (which are its terminal values) as well as the behaviours that the organization supports (which are its instrumental values). HFM-163 believes that for a NATO HQ to be able to attain its operative goals, its terminal cultural values must reflect flexibility and agility in its processes, yet stability in the organizational structure. Its instrumental cultural values should include trusting each other as well as being open to diversity and improvement orientation. The larger the degree to which the NATO HQ has developed these cultural values, the more it will support attaining the operative goals.

More detailed information about the HFM-163 Organizational Effectiveness model and its supporting theories will be found in the HFM-163 final report (NATO RTO HFM RTG 163 2012).

Methodological Aspects of the Kosovo Case Study

In 2010, the HFM-163 Organizational Effectiveness model was tested in a case study in KFOR HQ in Pristina, Kosovo. The purpose of this study was to investigate to what extent the input factors of the model had an effect on the operative goals, and also to find out which factors had the greatest effect on the goals. Both quantitative and qualitative data (that is, both questionnaires and interviews) were collected during four days by five members belonging to the HFM-163 team.

Instruments

Based on the model described in the previous section, a questionnaire and an interview protocol were created. The questionnaire consisted of 12 background questions (focusing on gender, age, nationality, number of previous deployments in a multinational HQ, role and total time of work in the HQ) and 60 questions relating to the input factors and operative goals of the model. For all questions (except the ones concerning background) the participants rated their level of agreement on a five-point Likert-type rating scale, ranging from *strongly disagree* to *strongly agree*. A sixth option, labelled *I don't know*, was also available if the participants could not answer a particular question.

The interview protocol was also created on the basis of the HFM-163 Organizational Effectiveness model. The protocol included background questions (similar to the questionnaire, except for two added questions about the interviewee's role and responsibility in the HQ) and questions that related to the input factors and operative goals. For each input factor question, the interviewee was asked how he/she perceived the situation in the HQ, what worked well/not so well, how this affected the daily work and, when possible, they were asked what the most critical factors affecting the specific issue were. The interviewees were encouraged to give examples whenever they could. The questions concerning the operative goals had a similar structure. The interviewees were asked how information sharing, decision-making and shared awareness works in the HQ; what worked well/not so well, and why; what the most critical factors to achieve these goals were; and also how they thought the factor at hand could be improved.

The interviews were designed to be semi-structured. The follow-up questions were, however, not posed to all participants; some extra questions were added when needed (depending on the answers of the interviewees).

Participants and Procedure

Questionnaire data were collected from 136 KFOR HQ staff members; more specifically, 103 military and 33 civilians. All hierarchical levels and departments of the staff were represented. The questionnaire data collection was organized into six sessions where 20–25 respondents participated each time. The questionnaire took about 15–20 minutes to complete.

The interviews were conducted with KFOR HQ personnel who held key positions in the staff, primarily at the Assistant Chief of Staff level, covering J1–J5, J8, HQ support group (HSG), military and civilian advisory team division (MCA) and joint information centre (JIC). All interviewees except two were military officers (Colonel or Lt Colonel). The interviewees were interviewed one at a time. Four persons from HFM-163 conducted the interviews in pairs. One person in the pair asked questions while the other documented the interview and posed additional questions if clarification was needed. Each interview lasted approximately 45–60 minutes. All interviews except one were audio-recorded. Before an interview started, the participants were informed that their participation was voluntary, that their anonymity would be protected; permission was also sought regarding the audio-recording of their involvement. All interviews were subsequently transcribed. Transcription was made into literary language and complete sentences, keeping the formulations and wordings used by the interviewees. Qualitative analyses of the interviews were performed by the four HFM-163 persons who had conducted the interviews. The interview answers were summarized into a table, so that the answers concerning each input factor or operative goal could be easily compared.

Results

Results were attained and analysed during two HFM-163 meetings, and also individually between meetings. FOI participated mainly in the analyses of interview data, so this chapter focuses primarily on the interview results, only briefly presenting questionnaire results. A complete description of the results can be found in the HFM-163 final report (NATO RTO HFM RTG 163 2012).

Questionnaire Findings

Many civilian employees (belonging to the staff) had been active since the beginning of the mission, that is, for about 10 years, whereas the military personnel rotated in cycles varying between 3 and 12 months. The civilian personnel, mainly contractors, were not part of the staff per se, therefore not our target audience. Since it was difficult to identify which of the civilian respondents actually were involved in the HQ staff work, all civilian questionnaires were excluded from the analyses. Consequently, the questionnaire results are deduced from 103 military respondents. A total of 60 questions relating to the input factors and operative goals were asked. The factor hierarchy and the factor centralization were combined into one in the analyses as a result of correlation analysis, where it turned out that there was a low correlation between the questions within each factor.

The results showed that the respondents believed that the KFOR HQ structure is hierarchical and centralized, rather than flat and decentralized. In addition to this, the respondents stated that within the staff there was a high degree of flexibility, effective leadership, trust, openness to diversity and improvement orientation; see Figure 10.2.

Furthermore, the results show that all operative goals and effectiveness were rated above average; see Figure 10.3.

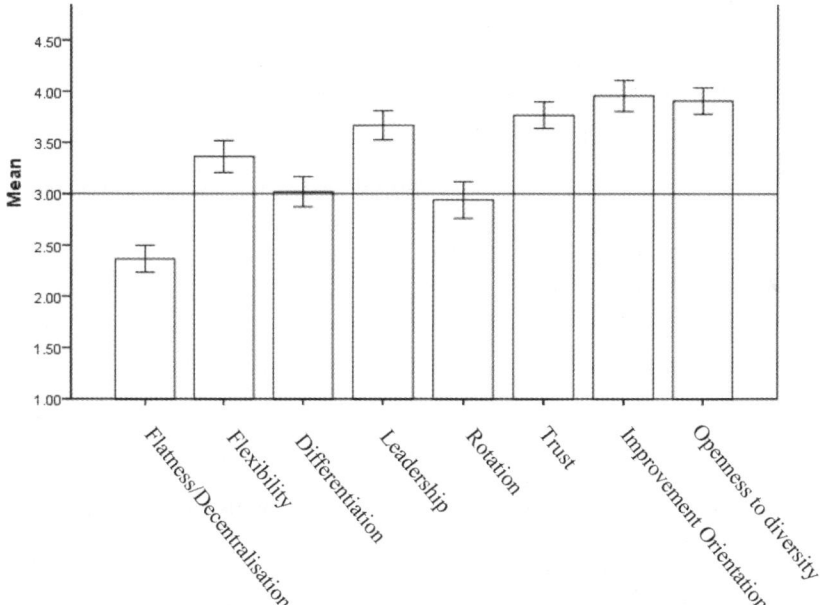

Figure 10.2   Descriptive statistics for ratings of input factors in KFOR HQ

Correlation analyses show that all input factors, except flat/decentralized structure, correlate positively with the operative goals, with coefficients between 0.11 and 0.65 and p-values that range from $p = 0.257$ (between the routines and perceived efficiency variables) to $p < 0.001$ (between the leadership and decision-making variables). Multiple regression analyses were calculated for every operative goal to test to what extent there was a significant statistical correlation between the input factors and the operative goal. The results are summarized here; for a more detailed description, see NATO RTO HFM RTG 163 (2012).

The results show, first, that flexibility, leadership effectiveness and trust had significant effects on decision-making. Secondly, leadership effectiveness and trust had significant effects on information sharing. Thirdly, flexibility, openness to change and trust had significant effects on information sharing. Fourthly – and finally – leadership effectiveness, openness to diversity and trust had significant effects on perceived organizational effectiveness. The significant effects between the input factors and operative goals are summarized in Figure 10.4.

Figure 10.4 shows that the two input factors leadership effectiveness and trust seem to have utmost effect on the operative goals.

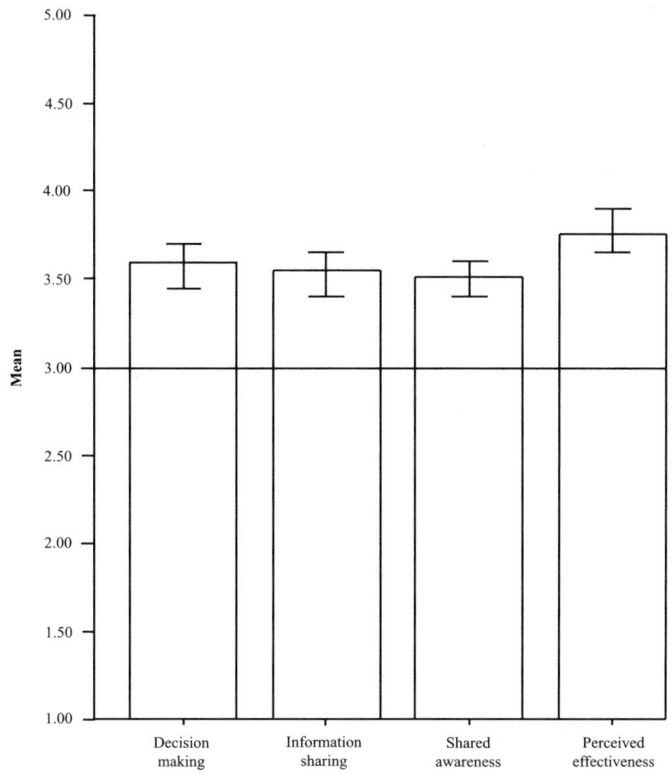

Figure 10.3   Descriptive statistics for operative goals and effectiveness

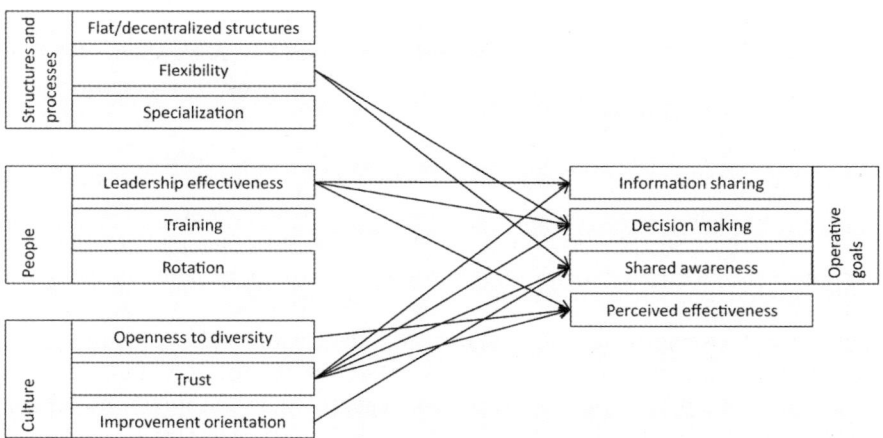

Figure 10.4   Summary of how the input factors affect the operative goals and perceived organizational effectiveness in KFOR HQ. (All relations in the figure are statistically significant)

Interview Findings

In this section, the results from the interviews are presented for every input factor and operative goal.

Organizational structure
The majority of the respondents believed that the HQ staff was organized in accordance with a so-called NATO J-structure. A few organizational changes had been made; for example, the branches J1 (personnel), J4 (logistics) and J-engineering had been merged into *one* branch for logistics and support. The general opinion from the interviewees was that the HQ had become flatter in its organizational structure than before (due to recent personnel reductions), although it was still perceived to be hierarchical. Those who perceived the HQ to be very hierarchical also stated that it was detrimental to work; that is, they thought the hierarchy made it more difficult to reach goals and coordinate efforts between branches, slowing down work as communication between branches was perceived as more difficult. The respondents believed that a flat organizational structure promotes all three operative goals (decision-making, information sharing and shared awareness).

Centralized and/or decentralized command processes
The results show that some of the interviewees thought that the command process was too centralized, while others argued that processes were too decentralized. Centralization was thought to be characteristic of how higher echelons of the HQ made decisions, while in day-to-day business command processes were viewed as more decentralized. Those who believed the HQ to be too centralized stated that it was causing 'bottlenecks' in information sharing and decision-making. Those with the opposite opinion stated that centralization is essential to ensure that political goals and strategies are met. Generally, the respondents thought that the HQ processes were centralized whereas the processes within their own branches were decentralized.

Flexibility
Most of the respondents thought that there was a high degree of flexibility within the HQ and, like the opinions about centralization, the interviewees perceived the flexibility to be higher within their own branches than in the HQ as a whole. Most of the SMEs believed that flexibility is crucial for an efficient HQ. However, some of the interviewees emphasized that even though flexibility is good, a clear structure is essential to keep focus within the staff. As regards the operative goals, the respondents thought that flexibility affects information sharing positively and that flexibility and decision-making interact; that is, decision-making is both affected by, and affects, the level of flexibility in the staff.

Specialized roles

All the interviewees believed that their roles in the HQ were specialized rather than overlapping. Specialization was generally viewed as something positive since it creates a clear division of work and allows a person to focus. However, some of the interviewees expressed a need for more overlap within the HQ since it creates a better understanding of the work conducted within other branches, facilitating information sharing and decision-making. Furthermore, one of the interviewees stated that overlapping roles are better than specialization when the HQ is not fully manned (due to vacancy or leave), since no one may be able to fill the role of the specialist who is absent.

Leadership effectiveness

The leadership of the KFOR HQ was described very positively by the interviewees. The leadership was characterized as 'comfortable', 'inclusive', 'open and friendly', 'respectful', 'supportive', 'professional' and 'effective'. Several respondents emphasized that the superiors are present (approachable) and listen to the opinions and suggestions of the subordinates before making decisions, something which was perceived to be important for good leadership. An effective leadership was believed to be of importance for all three operative goals.

Pre-deployment training

Since pre-deployment training is a national responsibility, the quantity and quality of training received differed between the interviewees. Some personnel had received national training only, while others received both national and multinational training. Most of the military interviewees had attended the two-week KFOR *Key Leader Training* course located at the KFOR HQ prior to their deployment. This was considered to be very good in that it made the start of the deployment easier; many of the respondents stated that this course should be mandatory. The need for training was considered to depend on personal experience (number of previous deployments) and whether the position was a staff or field position (field positions were perceived to require more training). The respondents stated that pre-deployment training creates a shared awareness of the roles and responsibilities within an HQ.

Personnel rotations and handover processes

Most interviewees had experienced a so called hand-over–take-over (HOTO) period of 1–2 weeks. Two weeks was considered sufficient; however, some thought that one week could be enough if the successor has experience from earlier deployments. A general opinion expressed by the interviewees was that the HOTO process together with the short rotation cycle reduces the effectiveness of the HQ by impeding institutional memory which, in turn, increases the amount of time it takes to learn the work. However, many believed that this 'dip' in efficiency could be minimized if the successors are well prepared and properly trained. One of the interviewees pointed out that the rotation process is part of every multinational HQ and instead of fighting the system, one should do one's best in a given situation. Frequent rotation was believed to be extra problematic for personnel in leading positions and also for positions where personal contacts with local actors are important. The interviewees thought those positions should be manned for at least a year. Some respondents believed that rotations could also be positive in that 'new eyes and new solutions' are brought into the HQ. In that way, rotations can have a positive effect on decision-making, but the rotations can also hamper the decision-making, especially when the decision-makers rotate. The interviewees believed that rotations, in a general sense, affect information sharing and shared awareness negatively.

Openness to diversity and multinationality
The interview questions relating to this input factor mainly focused on multinational aspects of the HQ. Most interviewees thought it was positive to have a multinational HQ since it gave the HQ more power. A multinational HQ is often viewed to be more neutral than a national HQ, and also has support from the international committee. Still, the interviewees generally believed that a multinational HQ is less effective than a national HQ. However, a common opinion was that multinationality in general is positive for decision-making because it brings different perspectives and solutions to problems. At the same time, information sharing and shared awareness can suffer from multinationality due to communication problems; that is, problems caused by varying language skills in English and other cultural differences.

Trust
Generally, the interviewees thought there was a high level of trust between the staff members in KFOR HQ. Two main perspectives on trust were represented. Some of the respondents expressed that they usually trusted other members of the HQ. Unless a person in some sense proved to be untrustworthy, the interviewees believed that the personnel in their respective positions had the right competences and qualifications to 'get the job done'. The other main opinion regarding trust was that this has to be earned or established, based on informal relationships and on daily work (products). Two of the interviewees talked about differences between organizational/official trust and individual trust. It appears that 'official trust is there from the beginning, while individual trust has to grow, like in families or friendships'. Since the question was not limited to a certain type of trust, a reason for these different opinions may be that some informants referred to official trust (based on organization, formal role, job description) while others to individual trust (related to persons). The respondents believed that there is an inverted relationship between trust and the operative goals. In other words, good information sharing and shared awareness creates trust.

Improvement orientation

To be improvement oriented is to allow initiatives to improve work, processes and routines, and this 'quality' has both advantages and disadvantages. It can, for example, lead to improvements – or generate mistakes. We asked the interviewees how improvement oriented they perceive the KFOR HQ to be.

The respondents were of different opinions on this matter. Some believed the HQ was improvement oriented; others did not share this view. The respondents believed that the KFOR HQ was improvement oriented since there was a will to improve the work *on all levels*. Some believed that ideas were generally accepted and that it was relatively easy to implement changes, especially on lower levels. Others believed that the rotation system, with its constant change of personnel, hampered the organization's ability to learn and improve since it lacks institutional memory. Just like trust, the interviewees believed that there was an inverted relationship between the input factor and the operative goals, where decision-making and shared awareness affects the ability to implement change.

Information sharing

Most of the interviewees thought that information was available and easily accessible in the KFOR HQ. One of the respondents stated that there is a lot of information available in the HQ and sharing the information is not the problem; rather, the challenge is to identify the *right* information. Therefore, the respondents believed that the critical issue about information sharing is to understand the information system (both technically and procedurally), that is, one needs to know where to look for information and how to get the relevant information. The interviewees also said that to enable information sharing, the personnel have to proactively look for information and be open to sharing information. To be able to do that, one must create an understanding of the information that other people need and where that information is available.

Decision-making

The interviewees thought that decision-making in KFOR HQ was efficient and that decisions were made at the right time. Decision processes were described as formal, in accordance with regulations, but still flexible. Some of the interviewees believed that the decision process was inclusive and that the decision-maker took input from others, whereas some of the respondents believed that the decision process was too centralized and should be delegated to the lower levels.

Shared awareness of tasks and responsibilities

All the interviewees thought that a shared awareness of tasks and responsibilities is essential for the KFOR HQ to be efficient. Knowing how work is distributed speeds up decision processes, enables reactivity and facilitates synchronization within the staff. However, there were differences in opinions as to whether or not there actually was a high degree of such an understanding in the KFOR

HQ. Training was believed to be a key factor in reaching a shared awareness for tasks and responsibilities.

Critical factors to improve effectiveness

At the end of each interview, the respondents had the opportunity to state what they thought were the most important aspects required to improve the effectiveness in the KFOR HQ. Some of the statements were (a) to give more responsibility and freedom to act to the lower levels in the chain of command; (b) to improve formal and informal information-sharing systems; (c) to centralize leadership; and (d) to organize motivational meetings where the commander meets with key staff, sharing his goals and acknowledging good efforts. The interviewees also emphasized the importance of manning positions for at least one year and spreading rotations more evenly during the year. To improve training and to send preparation packages to HQ personnel before starting deployment was also considered important, as was ensuring sufficient job experience and background. Other aspects included the understanding of operational planning processes, being proactive and making assessments about the future. The improvement of cultural interoperability was also mentioned. The last suggestion that was brought up was to interact more in the local community to facilitate a better understanding of the local population and generate a better understanding of the Kosovo environment.

Discussion and Concluding Remarks

After completing the KFOR HQ case study, we can conclude that the data collection went according to the initial plan. The questionnaire respondents covered all the functions in the staff, as well as all command levels. The turnout for the interviews was perhaps better than expected; only one person could not participate. It was, however, unfortunate that we had to disregard all the civilian respondents from the analyses of the questionnaire data. We should have ensured the identification of civilians who were part of our target group, as well as the ones that were not. Our ambition with the semi-structured interviews was to keep the questions relatively open so the interviewees would have the opportunity to present aspects of importance for organizational effectiveness that were not necessarily part of our model. However, the interview protocol did concern some specific questions about the factors in the model; consequently, there is a risk that the interviewees' responses were affected by that.

Nevertheless, it seems that the organizational effectiveness model developed by the HFM-163 team is valid. There is no evidence from the case study that indicate that any large modifications need to be made. The results show that some factors seem to be of more importance than others. There are also factors in the model that do not have much support from the case study; however, they are not contradicted. Thus there is not enough evidence to conclude that the model needs to be modified.

The results from the interviews also showed inverted dependencies: the operative goals were believed to influence the input factors. This was evident especially for the input factor *culture*. Shared awareness, good decision-making and well-functioning information sharing were said to create trust; decision-making was perceived to influence the possibility of implementing changes; and shared awareness was believed to lead to more openness to diversity.

Even though these dependencies are not shown in the current HFM-163 organizational effectiveness model, they are still important to take into consideration if – or when – an HQ is going to develop its organizational effectiveness.

The result of this research project has shown the need for comprehensive pre-deployment training for personnel who are to work in international headquarters. The results of the study can be of direct use for the Swedish Armed Forces in developing mission-specific training. The results also help to create a better understanding of the multinational environment, the challenges that mission personnel may encounter during their deployment and how these challenges can be met. Personnel in leading positions in a multinational headquarters will benefit from the results regarding leadership; factor knowledge is critical for the improvement of organizational effectiveness.

Finally, participating in a NATO research group of this kind is usually a cost-effective way of achieving interesting and new research results. A study such as the one described in this chapter would be costly to conduct by a single nation. However, by bringing together researchers from different nations, NATO research groups can gather expertise from different countries and accomplish magnificent results out of individual efforts.

References

Daft, R.L. (1998). *Organization, Theory and Design*. 6th edition. Cincinnati: South-Western College Publishing.

Essens, P., Vogelaar, A., Mylle, J., Blendell, C., Paris, C., Halpin, S. and Baranski, J. (2005). *Military Command Team Effectiveness: Model and Instrument for Assessment and Improvement*. Technical Report AC/323(HFM-087)TP/59.

Galbraith, J.R. (2002). *Designing Organizations. An Executive Guide to Strategy, Structure, and Processes*. San Francisco: Jossey-Bass Publishers.

Gilbert, T.F. (1996). *Human Competence: Engineering Worthy Performance (Tribute Edition)*. Washington DC: International Society for Performance Improvement.

Jones, G.R. (2004). *Organizational Theory, Design, and Change. Text and Cases*. Upper Saddle River, NJ: Pearson Education.

NATO RTO (2011). NATO RTO website. Available at http://ww.rto.nato.int [accessed 1 October 2011].

NATO RTO HFM RTG 163. (2012). *Improving Organizational Effectiveness in Coalition Operations*. Final report RTO-TR-HFM-163 AC/323(HFM-163) TP/476.

Peters, T. and Waterman, R.H. Jr. (1982). *In Search of Excellence*. New York, London: Harper & Row.

Porter, M.E. (1996). What is strategy? *Harvard Business Review*, 74(6), 61–78.

Chapter 11
Agility in Command and Control – Functional Models of Cognition

B.J.E. Johansson

Introduction

Functional models of cognition can be used to explain command and control agility. However, it is necessary to point to generic cognitive functions that must be part of any command and control system presenting agility. As research stands today, previous command and control models have not included the notion of agility. Agility is the ability to transform an organization into the type of organization that is most appropriate to the circumstances at hand. Simply adapting any current command and control model is therefore problematic as this rarely explains (a) the self-monitoring required to recognize the need for change, (b) the ability to, as it were, move functions across structures, (c) how context(s) affect(s) performance and (d) the proactive behaviour demanded for agility (for example goal production, adaption).

Functional models of cognition, on the other hand, explain why an organism behaves in a purposeful manner and therefore also have the potential to explain why a command and control organization can do that too. Models of command and control systems (in a functional sense) often resemble models of cognition, cognitive agents or general models of goal-driven behaviour (Taylor 2002; Stanton et al. 2001) since the command and control system, as an organism, tries to adapt to its environment. Focusing on behaviour, a living organism and a command and control system are not entirely different since they demand the same set of basic functions in order to survive. Examples of such functions are perception (intelligence), decision-making, tools for interacting with or affecting the environment (for example military units); all in all the fundamental properties of a system presenting cognition.

A cognitive system can be described as a system that can 'modify its behaviour on the basis of experience so as to achieve specific anti-entropic ends' (Hollnagel and Woods 2005: 22). Achieving anti-entropic ends in complex and dynamic environments equals having the requisite variety to do so. This suggests that such a system must be able to formulate goals and present both reactive (feedback-driven) *and* proactive (feed-forward-driven) behaviour. This is also a requirement for agile command and control systems (Alberts et al. 2010), as command and control agility is intended to, for example, be a way to increase the variety of a given command and control system. In the following, it is argued that a command and control system that can reconfigure its structure concerning some basic functions *is* command and control agile. Such a process puts demands on individuals, organization and technology relating to a given command and control system.

There are several models available that explain reactive and proactive behaviour, although most models are essentially feedback driven. Perhaps the most commonly used model for describing command and control is the Observe, Orient, Decide, Act (OODA) loop as described by Boyd. It has been adopted and (re)interpreted over the years, most recently by Brehmer (2006) in the shape of the DOODA loop, that is, *dynamic* OODA. The 'heir' models of the OODA loop are all feedback-driven, cybernetic models based on the idea that speed is imperative in a conflict situation, as the side that is able to act before the other will also be the winning side. Decision quality is naturally also important, as is the capacity to turn decision to action. Brehmer acknowledges the practical difficulties of this by introducing Clausewitz's notion of *friction* into the DOODA loop, illustrating that even the best plan may be hampered by unforeseen events when turned into practice (Clausewitz 1997; Brehmer 2006).

Of relevance, and also hinted above, is that problems emerge when models similar to OODA are used to understand the new, updated, term 'command and control agility'. It should be noted that command and control agility involves something *more* than simply responding in a timely and efficient manner to changes, namely the ability to observe the organization in relation to the environment, and also to recognize the necessity to make changes to its command and control approach.

There is a difference between agility and command and control agility (Alberts et al. 2010). Agility concerns the ability of a military organization (or a joint force) to cope with and reach their goals in a complex and dynamic environment, very much in agreement with the definition of a cognitive system presented above. Command and control agility, moreover, concerns the ability to do so by changing the command and control approach, that is, involves the ability to recognize and progress to a command and control approach that is appropriate for a situation as it evolves. How a command and control system positions itself in relation to other types of command and control systems can be discussed by placing it into the command and control approach space.

The command and control approach space was presented in Alberts et al. (2010), more specifically as having three dimensions: allocation of decision rights, distribution of information *and* interaction patterns among entities (see Figure 11.1). An approach space is not intended as a tool showing that Edge command and control (the 'top' level command and control approach in Figure 11.1) by necessity is preferred to a traditional hierarchical approach. Alberts et al. emphasized, instead, the need to use an approach that fits the challenge of a current mission, leaning on Ashby's idea of *requisite variety* (Ashby 1956). The fact that a command and control system has the capacity to move (with)in a part of an approach space is referred to as the *maturity level*. Alberts et al. (2010) argue the following:

In establishing a strategy for an entity, it is important that an appropriate C2 [command and control] maturity level is selected; one that will allow the entity to function appropriately in the mix of situations and circumstances that the entity will be involved in over time. Excess maturity (C2 approach options that are not required for the set of circumstances envisioned) comes at a cost, while deficient maturity (not being able to utilise the appropriate approach when it is required) may result in failures to cope successfully. We describe the specific maturity level that fits an entity's mission space as Requisite C2 Maturity. [p. xxii]

However, the movement between different command and control approaches is not sufficient in itself for the achievement of requisite variety; a command and control system must also be able to monitor itself (its own organization/ system) *as well as* the environment in which it operates; the relation between the two essentially decides if and when a change in command and control approach is needed. Self-awareness and context are thus central components of a model describing a system that presents command and control agility. A working model of this type may look like that in Figure 11.2. There certainly were computers capable of performing parallel execution of programs at the time, but most models of cognition still described neat, ordered sequences – with some notable exceptions; see, for example, Neisser (1976).

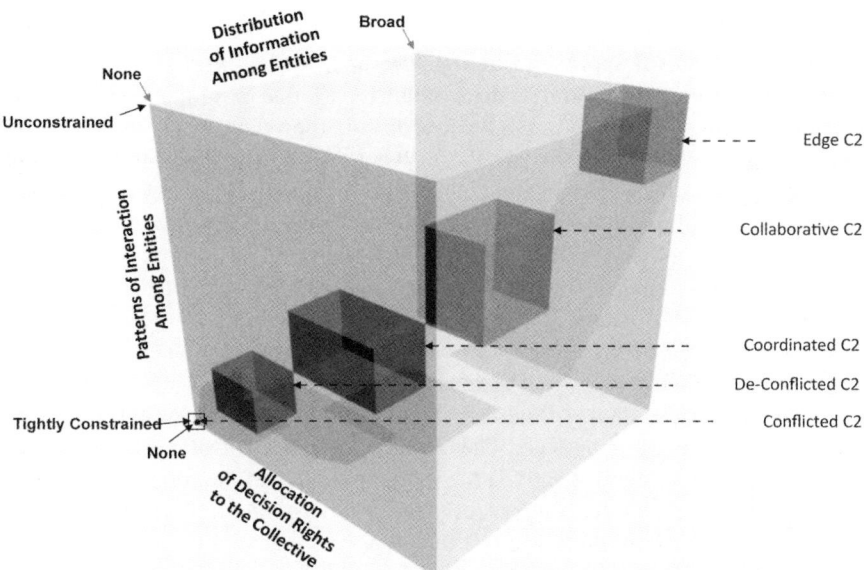

Figure 11.1   The command and control approach space
Source: Alberts et al. (2010).

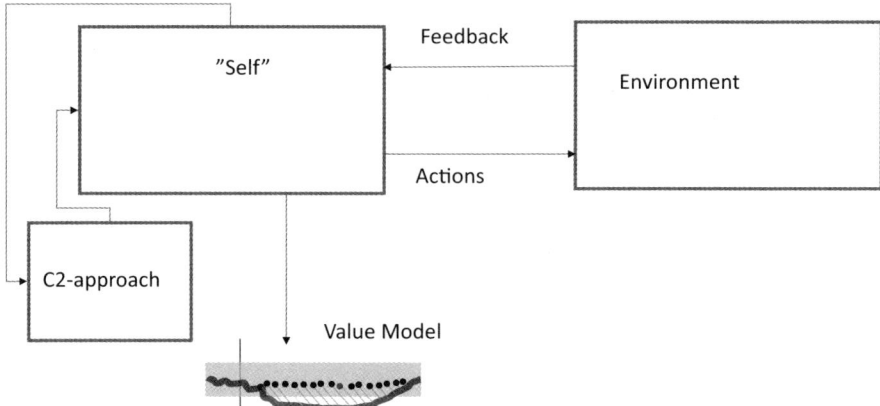

Figure 11.2   A possible model of a command and control system presenting command and control agility

The model presented in Figure 11.2 depicts a system that compares the value model with the feedback it gets from actions taken in its current, existing environment. The value model is a description of the desired state that the command and control system intends to create or maintain both in terms of self and environment. In the case of command and control agility, the means for doing so is to adjust its own command and control approach, or adapt another command and control approach (if this is possible). The number of possible command and control approaches that a command and control system can take constitutes the command and control maturity of that command and control system; the area of the command and control approach space in which the command and control system has the competence and equipment to operate. This implies that the command and control system somehow must be self-aware; that it must be able to monitor and reflect upon its own behaviour in relation to the environment, a kind of meta-cognitive skill using the analogy of a cognitive system presented above. Also, the environment, the context of the system, is a driving factor that needs more attention than it receives in most models of command and control systems. After all, it is the relation between the self and the state of the environment that creates demands for agility.

A model like the one in Figure 11.2 may serve as a conceptual model for explaining the relation between the command and control system and the environment, but it does not explain the inner processes of the self; functions that comprise the ability to act purposefully in an environment. Therefore, models are needed that can explain how context(s) shapes the behaviour of an organism/system and how an organism/system works. In this regard, this chapter presents the movement towards a general model of an agile system.

Theoretical Background

All control activity – or behaviour – exists in a context that in turn shapes the same activity/behaviour in a reciprocal manner (Neisser 1976; Vygotsky 1978; Suchman 1987; Hutchins 1995; Hollnagel and Woods 2005). As models are generally based on idealized versions of activities, they tend to miss, be incapable of describing, the details that any practitioner will recognize as important, especially when understanding why something works – or not. As mentioned above, Clausewitz used the notion *friction* to explain the small things that differentiate reality from a planned course of action in a military context; an observation as valid today as it was 150 years ago. What friction actually illustrates is the human limitation of prediction, especially when complex organizations such as the military are involved. The mere number of interacting humans and the technology they use creates an enormous coordination task. In the military example, there are also one or several antagonists, who actively try to control the behaviour of the command and control system. Neither of these two contextual factors is normally part of command and control models.

Cognitive Systems Engineering

The field of *cognitive systems engineering* (CSE) originates from a different context than most of the models and theories of military command and control, although it shares some of the problems that command and control modelling and understanding face today. CSE was, to some extent, the result of the problems associated with modelling human performance using the concepts and methods that were prevailing at the time (the early 1980s), but also a consequence of the increasing complexity of socio-technical systems, resulting from applied computerization in the form of decision-support systems and information technology. There was (still is) a 'self-reinforcing complexity cycle' in progress which works according to 'the law of stretched systems' (as suggested by Hirschhorn; Hollnagel and Woods 2005). The cycle implies that complexity in socio-technical systems is bound to increase since more and more advanced technology is used to enhance performance, increasing the internal complexity of the system itself. With increased complexity follow heightened levels of unpredictability, even if system performance as such becomes more stable; outcomes of failure are simply more difficult to predict. Further, CSE was a response to the inability of the modelling approaches dominant at the time to predict performance. When the original CSE paper by Hollnagel and Woods was published in 1983, the common approach to modelling cognition, hence behaviour, was to use models based on assumptions of information processing. The analogy of the human brain as computer machinery created sequential models mostly focused on response rather than anticipation, structure rather than function; most importantly, treating context as something indirect, mediated, via input to the system (Hollnagel and Woods 2005). It should be noted that a similar model is part of Alberts (2011). The impact of situational features and the environment in which a cognitive agent acts was usually not recognized in the case of modelling. The similarities between the commonly referenced technological revolution and the somewhat problematic ways of modelling within the current command and control domain can hardly be neglected. The concurrent technical revolution presents different problems, and concerns networking rather than computational power, but the modelling problems largely suffer from the same difficulties as cognitive modelling did in 1983.

In what way, then, can CSE help us to understand agility? One suggestion here is to look into some of the modelling attempts that have been made in CSE, especially those concerning contextual models. These have been developed to illustrate how a human, or any 'cognitive system', performs in a specific context. These models also describe some basic functions that must be fulfilled by any system presenting both feedback- and feed-forward-driven behaviour. Once this is accomplished, we must examine how such functions may exist in parallel in a military organization.

Contextual Control Model

The *contextual control model* (COCOM) is an attempt to describe control as a result of competence and knowledge about a current situation, context(s) and time pressure. According to Taylor (2002), the COCOM is intended to be applicable to 'a range of systems, including individuals, joint cognitive systems and complex socio-technical systems'. The model itself contains four *control modes* that a system may attain: scrambled, opportunistic, tactical and strategic mode. According to Hollnagel (1998), time is one of the most important determinants for control, and for judgements of the control mode that a current cognitive system can be in. Scrambled mode implies the lowest form of control, presenting a behaviour that is irrational, signified by seemingly random actions. Opportunistic control is based on reactive control, where response is driven by salient environmental features. Tactical control is orderly and is signified by being proactive to some extent, but primarily relies on known strategies and heuristics. Recognition-primed decision-making, as described by Klein (1998), can be interpreted as a mix of opportunistic and tactical control. Strategic control is orderly and anticipates higher-level goals. Elaborate planning is a part of strategic control.

Hollnagel has also proposed a *basic cyclical model* (Figure 11.3), founded on Neisser's perceptual cycle (Neisser 1976; Hollnagel 1993, 1998). The basic cyclical model is similar to, for example, the OODA loop, but is signified by two important differences: (a) the explicit presence of a target system and (b) the presence of feedback disturbances, indicating that it may be difficult – even impossible – to interpret whether the outcome of an event is the effect of own actions or some form of external intervention.

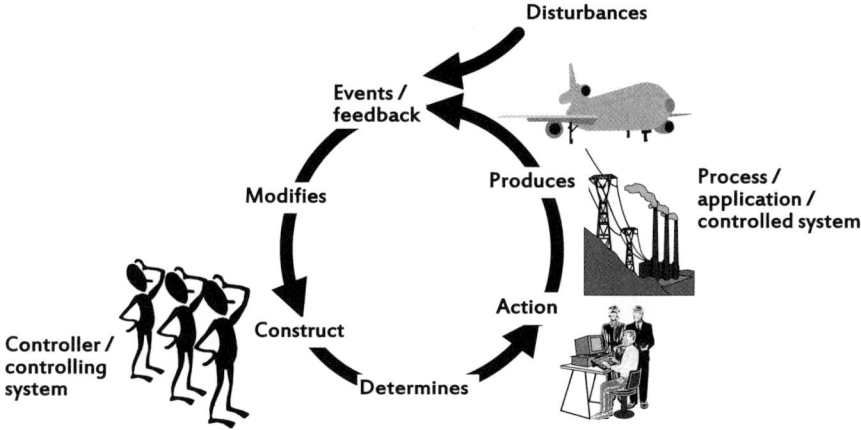

Figure 11.3   The basic cyclical model
Source: Hollnagel (1998).

The COCOM has some important implications for agility as it focuses on and thereby emphasizes the importance of time and time pressure. Such time aspects should be part of any agility model since available time is essential for the understanding of whether a command and control system will be able to respond to external events, and/or if there will be enough time to progress from one command and control approach to another. Secondly, the COCOM emphasizes the difficulties of interpreting surrounding events and also happenings within the self. There are always disturbances to this process, not only in the form of noise (making it difficult to interpret transmitted signals) but also in terms of ambiguity when reasoning about cause and effect. In war, or warlike situations, it is often difficult to judge if observed events are caused by own actions, other actors' interventions or mere coincidence. This decision is perhaps more complicated to make for complex endeavours where battles may preferably be fought in political arenas. In such situations, even minor military actions may create extensive, unpredictable outcomes in terms of political or societal instability.

According to the COCOM, the ability to interpret and to respond adequately to feedback largely depends on a controller's competence. Context(s), available time and competence *together* decide the possible control mode a system may reach. This statement is valid for any system trying to control something, and should therefore also be part of a model of an agile system. What the COCOM does not explain, however, are the basic functions required for control. More importantly, the COCOM does not explain how proactive behaviour (for example, goal formulation) actually emerges.

The Extended Control Model

The *extended control model* (ECOM; Hollnagel et al. 2003; Hollnagel and Woods 2005) identifies patterns in control behaviour on the basis of performance. It is, like OODA and similar models, built on feedback processes, which underline dynamics between perceiving and acting. ECOM also involves proactive control functions. The ECOM provides means for identification of patterns in activities performed on parallel, interacting levels in a command and control system. In detail, the ECOM describes performance in relation to activities on four different, goal-related, levels (see Figure 11.4).

First, there is *targeting*, a controller's or controlling system's anticipations of events in future plans and goals. Short- and long-term goals are set up and given priority, thus affecting lower levels. Secondly, there is *monitoring*, implying that a controller keeps track of an environment and its actions, producing plans out of feedback from lower levels *and* expectations from higher levels. Generated plans are then used by regulating and tracking loops. Thirdly, we find *regulating*, meaning that resources are managed in relation to goals and environmental changes, often involving a number of tracking sub-loops. Lastly, there is *tracking*, performance of feedback tasks controlled by higher levels' goals and targets.

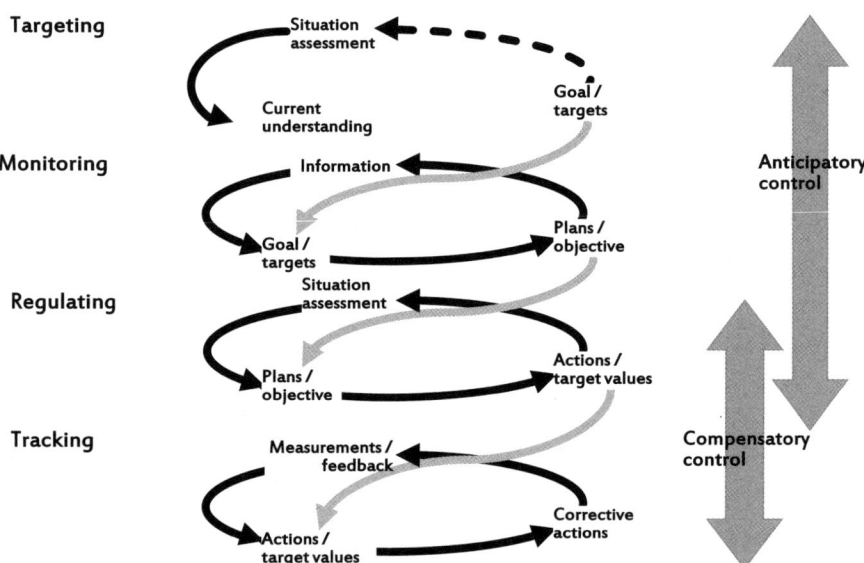

Figure 11.4   The extended control model
Source: Hollnagel and Woods (2005).

According to the ECOM, performance takes place simultaneously on concurrent loops of activity, that is, at the same time and interconnected with regard to goals – but within different time frames. One fundamental assumption is that this is valid both for individuals and more complex socio-technical systems such as command and control systems. Their coupling is represented in the way a higher levels' output serves as input for the subordinate level in the form of objectives. Thereby, a direct interdependence between objectives/plans and activities is outlined. Different types of assessments are required at every level, exemplified through activities.

A command and control system must be in control of all loops at the same time; dependencies between the levels must have appropriate interfaces to each other, otherwise the input from a higher loop to a lower one (in the form of objectives) is not appropriately acted upon (and vice versa). It is, however, also possible to reduce or to halt activities on one or several levels to cope with occurring, mutually affecting, disturbances. This applies to many cases, for example driving, where a tricky driving situation can force a driver to stop navigating and to focus more on manoeuvring, thus avoiding an accident at the cost of continuing in the wrong direction. The ECOM clearly gives opportunities to discuss proactive behaviour through its introduction of targeting and monitoring loops. It is a fact that, for example, the DOODA loop (Brehmer 2006) also includes a planning function, but in this particular model, planning is not a parallel activity, rather something continuously revised through environmental feedback, thus merely an instance of feedback control. This implies that continuous planning cannot be an option if the logic of the DOODA model is followed.

The ECOM and Command and Control Agility

The ECOM is useful for explaining proactive *and* reactive behaviour, as well as a mixture of the two. The model can actually also explain why an individual or organization is adaptive, that is, changes its behaviour in the light of earlier experience. Such experience can be immediate, as in the case of responding to current events, but also long term, based on reflection upon past events (Kontogiannis 2010). Specifically, the targeting loop provides this possibility since this loop creates new goals for lower-level functions. Depending on the level of analysis in a command and control organization, high-level goals may be given by a higher-level command, but an organization/system must also be able to produce goals on its own. As stated above, the model is based on four parallel interacting loops. These loops should be seen as basic functions of the cognitive system to which they belong. It is reasonable to suggest that any system that can be considered to be autonomous must have these functions in order to survive in a dynamic and complex environment. As stated earlier, an agile system is defined similarly to a cognitive system, and the ECOM is intended to be a general model of a cognitive system; it may also be a model of agility.

Which type of additional features does the ECOM present in relation to other models of agility/command and control? First, it describes cognition/command and control as a parallel activity, something that most other models do not. Virtually all other models are described in terms of sequences or logical if–then processes. Although many command processes can be described accordingly, most individuals with experience from the command and control domain would agree that this is not the case in the real world. Most importantly, it is not the case for the envisioned agile organization. Secondly, it focuses on *function* (rather than structure). Although these two concepts are interdependent, many benefits can be gained by focusing on functional models as points of departure. Brehmer (2006, 2007) – see also Rasmussen (1986), Rasmussen and Petersen (1994) – makes a strong argument for the use of functional models, as functions (the 'what' of a model) are the basis for the design, or manifestation, of a system. Brehmer further suggests that analysis should be carried out on two levels, the functional level *and* the product level (the 'how'). Functional analysis is analytical and examines the functions needed to fulfil a purpose. The product level is more constrained, shaped by organization, methods, processes, technology and so on, thus representing the outcomes of manifested functions, or how the functions actually work in reality. The connection between function and manifestation is also a powerful analytical tool, especially in the light of command and control agility, this being the ability to take on the organizational form/structure that is most appropriate for a current problem or situation.

Another way of putting it is to say that the command and control system can reconfigure itself in such a way that the distribution of resources between the ECOM functions fit the problem at hand. An unpredicted disturbance requires more resources to the 'lower', reactive functions; during calmer periods, resources should be spent on 'higher' levels, such as targeting and monitoring. Consider, for example, the characteristics of hierarchical organizations in comparison to edge organizations. A hierarchical organization is designed for executing well-formulated plans, while an edge organization is able to respond more quickly to environmental changes. Turning from theory to practice or reality, there are systems that already exhibit command and control agility. For example, organizations designed to face highly unpredictable environments, such as crisis management units or the rescue services, exhibit such ability. In everyday situations, they function as hierarchy, but in stressed situations they have the ability to join larger collectives and transfer functions across roles and organizations.

ECOM and the Military Context

One of the drawbacks of the ECOM in comparison with its predecessor the COCOM/basic cyclic model, at least in a graphical depiction, is that the target system is implicit. Considering a military context, this becomes a problem. In a military situation, there are actually at least two cognitive systems/command and control systems trying to control each other. Both of them exist in an operating context where they exchange actions with each other and the environment.

Disturbance
(Noise, non–related information, service failures etc.)

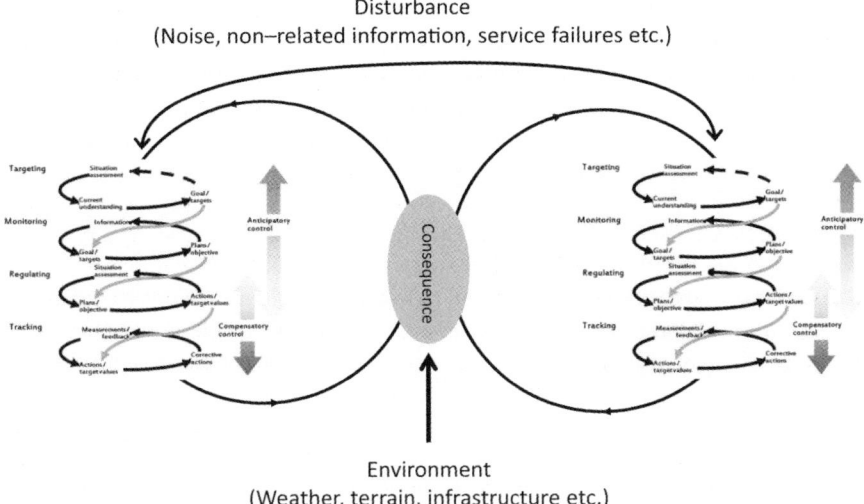

Environment
(Weather, terrain, infrastructure etc.)

Figure 11.5   The ECOM in a military context

The progress of the interaction is thus partly a product of the interaction between them, but also of environmental disturbances, which may be more or less dynamic. This brings us to a model that not only includes the system itself, but also contextual features and enemies. According to the law of requisite variety, a controlling system must present at least the same variation as the system to be controlled to remain in control. Having the ability to move within the command and control approach space is one way of increasing variety. A military scenario always includes at least two hostile actors, meaning that the concept of requisite variety is pointless without at least making assumptions about the variety of both parts in a conflict. If we assume that an entire organization/system is represented by the functions of the ECOM, we find a model that looks like Figure 11.5.

The model is naturally simplistic in that it only presents some basic functions, and not many of the fundamental structural components of military activity, such as resources in terms of forces/platforms, sensor capacity, reserves and so on. The possible agility (and effectiveness) of an organization or system is naturally also affected by these factors. The functions must hence be mapped to the structural (manifest) components in order to be used beyond conceptual discussions. For example, the ability to monitor depends on what kind of sensors and information paths exist in the organization(s) (as suggested by the command and control approach space). The ability to regulate depends on the available tools in terms of units, equipment and so forth that the command and control system has access to. The relation between structure (how individuals, technology and authority is organized) and function is thus of utmost importance when considering agility. For example, in a traditional hierarchical organization, only specialist or top nodes have access to sensor information. Decision rights are distributed top-down, creating dependencies between all actors (see the command and control approach space, Figure 11.1). In terms of the ECOM functions, higher-level cognitive functions (goal setting and other forms of tactical or strategic decision-making) have structurally been positioned at the top of the organization in order to increase control and predictability in terms of unit behaviour at the lower parts of the hierarchy (that perform the regulating and tracking functions). Mission tactics is one acknowledged exception to this, where subordinate units are given freedom in accomplishing their task. This does, however, also create demands on subordinate units to have the capacity to set goals and act independently. In an organization where power is more evenly distributed, like in an Edge organisation (see the command and control approach space, Figure 11.1), control may flow in the structure depending on how the situation evolves; that is the concept that brings viability to Edge organizations. This can also be seen in emergency management (at least in Sweden), where the commander at the emergency site is the person with highest decision power or authority. If he/she moves away from the site, the next person takes over command, based on the straightforward idea that the commander nearest the situation is the one best prepared and/or skilled to make decisions. In such a situation, the unit of analysis from a structural point of view may change over time as functions move between individuals and organizations. This has been shown and discussed by Aminoff et al. (2007) and in Trnka and Johansson (2009, 2011).

Discussion

The COCOM shows how context, competence and time shape the behaviour of an individual or an organization when trying to control a situation. The ECOM expands COCOM by describing some basic functions that must be fulfilled by any system that acts in a purposeful manner. In this chapter, it has been suggested that if a command and control system is to be considered agile, it must be able to reconfigure itself in such a way that the distribution of resources between the ECOM functions fit the problem at hand. This can be done by making transitions between different configurations, or command and control approaches. Transitions in responsibility and control, within or even between organizations, always create a vulnerable situation since it is both resource and time demanding to carry them out. While changing from one system state to another, the system exists in a form of limbo. Disturbances during transition may have severe consequences since the function under transition probably suffers from poor performance.

State Transitions and Coping

Yet, if we consider the relation between function and structure, such transitions constitute the core functionality of an agile system or organization (as pointed out, for example, in the command and control maturity space); the ability to move functions across structures as well as the ability to change structures. To develop methods and implementations for the support of transitions, as well as developing monitoring tools that can detect the need for a coming transition, is thus essential. In many cases, such preparations exist, but when concerned with inter-organizational work, preparations are indeed often absent. The interface between organizations may be non-existent or poorly defined, thus demanding both time and resources to be established (Johansson and Persson 2009). A particularly important question is how organizational/system performance is affected if a transition fails, that is, if responsibility or other necessary information is unclear, even lost. The relation between function and structure is apparent when such transitions are studied.

Trnka and Johansson (2011) study how functions move over time between different organizations and roles in a joint crisis management operation. An important point made by that work is that when trying to understand a highly adaptive organization, it is necessary to realize that it is not an entity with a given shape and function; rather, it takes its form through adaptations to unfolding situations, according to constraints set by organizational, social and technological structures, as well as operational missions. The degree to which structures are interoperable and flexible is what makes it possible to move a function. *Structural agility* thus enables *functional agility*, which is precisely what is strived for.

As shown in Figure 11.2, agility not only depends on the ability to change, but also on the ability of the self to recognize the need and be willing to do so. The resistance to change in an organization is as important a factor (when considering agility) as the willingness to do so. Lundberg et al. (2012) refer to such resistance as the *stiffness* of an organization or team. We thus need to better understand structural and functional agility, and what it means for individuals, technology and organizations. People must be willing to make the transitions, take on different roles in different situations and share information with others when needed. This puts demands on leadership, trust, communicative skills and so on (Johansson and Persson 2009), so the knowledge has to be incorporated in the training of agile forces. Technology must allow reconfiguration, interoperability, redundancy and so on. An organization becomes a special type of problem as it, by definition, becomes volatile in the sense that it is subject to change. It may be described in terms of predefined structures (hierarchies, collaborative entities or edge), as suggested in the command and control approach space, but it may just as well take on other forms or mixtures of different approaches. This is evident when considering collectives where several different organizations with different command and control approaches participate. The future challenge is to find ways of training people and developing technologies to enable agility.

References

Alberts, D.S. (2011). *The Agility Advantage: A Survival Guide for Complex Enterprises and Endeavors*. Washington DC: CCRP.

Alberts, D.S., Huber, R. and Moffat, J. (2010). *NATO NEC C2 Maturity Model*. Washington DC: CCRP Publication Series.

Aminoff, H., Johansson, B. and Trnka, J. (2007). Understanding communication in emergency response. In *Proceedings of the EAM 2007*. Copenhagen, Denmark.

Ashby, W.R. (1956). *An Introduction to Cybernetics*. London: Methuen & Co.

Brehmer, B. (2006). One loop to rule them all. In *Proceedings of the 11th ICCRTS*. Cambridge, UK, 26 September 2006. Available at http://www.dodccrp. org/events/11th_ICCRTS/iccrts_main.html [accessed 14 February 2014].

Brehmer, B. (2007). Understanding the functions of C2 is the key to progress. *The International C2 Journal*, 1(1), 211–32.

Clausewitz, C. (1997). *On War*. Ware: Wordsworth Editions Limited.

Hollnagel, E. (1993). Models of cognition: Procedural prototypes and contextual control. *Le Travail humain*, 56(1), 27–51.

Hollnagel, E. (1998). Context, cognition and control. In Y. Waern (ed.), *Co-operation in Process Management. Cognition and Information Technology*. London: Taylor & Francis.

Hollnagel, E., Nåbo, A. and Lau, I.V. (2003). A systemic model of driver-in-control. In *Proceedings of the Second International Driving Symposium on Human Factors in Driver Assessment, Training and Vehicle Control*. Park City, Utah, 86–91.

Hollnagel, E. and Woods, D.D. (2005). *Joint Cognitive Systems. Foundations of Cognitive Systems Engineering*. Boca Raton, FL: Taylor & Francis.

Hutchins, E. (1995). *Cognition in the Wild*. Cambridge, MA: MIT Press.

Johansson, B. and Persson, P.-A. (2009). Reduced uncertainty through human communication in complex environments. *Cognition, Technology & Work*, 11, 205–14.

Klein, G. (1998). *Sources of Power*. Cambridge, MA: MIT Press.

Kontogiannis, T. (2010). Adapting plans in progress in distributed supervisory work: Aspects of complexity, coupling and control. *Cognition, Technology & Work*, 12, 103–18.

Lundberg, J., Törnqvist, E. and Nadjm-Tehrani, S. (2012). Resilience in sensemaking and control of emergency response. *International Journal of Emergency Response*, 8(2), 99–122.

Neisser, U. (1976). *Cognition and Reality: Principles and Implications of Cognitive Psychology*. San Francisco: W.H. Freeman.

Rasmussen, J. (1986). *Information Processing and Human–Machine Interaction: An Approach to Cognitive Engineering*. New York: North-Holland.

Rasmussen, J. and Petersen, A.M. (1994). *Cognitive Systems Engineering*. New York: Wiley.

Stanton, N.A., Ashleigh, M.J., Roberts, A.D. and Zu, F. (2001). Testing Hollnagel's contextual control model: Assessing team behaviour in a human supervisory control task. *Journal of Cognitive Ergonomics*, 5(1), 21–33.

Suchman, L. (1987). *Plans and Situated Action*. New York: Cambridge University Press.

Taylor, R. (2002). *Capability, Cognition and Autonomy*. Keynote address to the NATO RTO Human Factors and Medicine Panel Symposium, HFM-084/ SY009, Warsaw, Poland, 7–9 October 2002.

Trnka, J. and Johansson, B. (2009). Collaborative command and control practice: Adaptation, self-regulation and supporting behaviour. *Int. J. Information Systems for Crisis Response and Management*, 1(2), 47–67.

Trnka, J. and Johansson, B. (2011). Resilient emergency response: Supporting flexibility and improvisation in collaborative command and control. In M.E. Jennex (ed.), *Crisis Response and Management and Emerging Information Systems: Critical Applications*. Hershey, PA: IGI Global, 112–38.

Vygotsky, L.S. (1978). *Mind in Society: The Development of Higher Psychological Processes*. Cambridge, MA: Harvard University Press.

Chapter 12

Conclusions

P. Berggren, S. Nählinder and E. Svensson

This book offers a description of the current state of command and control research in settings where sample sizes are small, opportunities are few and resources are limited. Special attention is given to the development of command and control research methods to meet current and coming needs. The authors also look forward towards a future where effective assessment of command and control abilities are even more crucial, for instance in agile organizations.

The individual chapter authors approach these issues in different ways. Some chapters discuss methodological aspects, others deal with theoretical concerns, and some with the empirical examples.

The purpose of command and control research is to improve the command and control process and make it more effective while still saving time and money. The research methods have to be chosen carefully to be effective and simple, yet provide results of high quality. In Chapters 4 and 7 it was explained how dynamic situations can be assessed and analysed, and examples were provided on how dynamic assessment can be performed.

Methodological concerns are a major consideration when working under such circumstances, and these considerations were dealt with in Chapters 2 and 3. Wikberg (Chapter 3) also showed how to perform iterative development cycles, and thus satisfy the demand to quickly deliver results from the research process. In Chapter 8, Berggren took another approach in dealing with methodological concerns and illustrated the development of an instrument for assessing shared understanding in teams.

In Chapter 9, examples are given on how field research experimentation can be quick, simple and effective, even though sample sizes are small and resources are limited. In such conditions, empirical data often need to be collected using measures and procedures that are minimally intrusive. Chapter 10 described how a field study is performed in an international context with officers in theatre.

Trnka and Woltjer discussed differences and similarities between civil and military command and control in Chapter 6.

Chapter 5 gives a description of the current state of international command and control research in relation to the concept of agility; Chapter 11 continued the theme of agility to discuss the next steps.

In summary, this book has shown how command and control studies can be performed in field settings characterized by dynamic and complex situations where opportunities are rare, money is decreasing and access to resources (personnel) is limited. We also explain how complex command and control situations can be assessed using dynamic methods and advanced statistical procedures. The importance of the involvement of end users is stressed and examples of how the stakeholders and end users can be involved in the command and control research process are provided. The relationship to command and control in emergency and disaster management is elaborated upon.

The command and control assessment methods and examples within this book provide tools for dealing with a changing world.

Index